The Encyclopedia of Medical Tests

Cathey Pinckney
and Edward R. Pinckney, M.D.

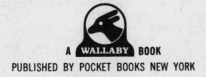

A WALLABY BOOK

PUBLISHED BY POCKET BOOKS NEW YORK

"*Listen* to the patient;
he is trying to tell you the diagnosis."
SIR WILLIAM OSLER

NOTICE

This book is not a manual for self-diagnosis. A physician should be consulted for proper interpretation of test results and diagnoses of medical conditions.

See the Introduction for important information on the significance of normal and abnormal test values.

POCKET BOOKS, a Simon & Schuster division of
GULF & WESTERN CORPORATION
1230 Avenue of the Americas, New York, N.Y. 10020

ISBN: 0-671-79057-9

First Wallaby printing September, 1978

1 2 3 4 0 9 8

Trademarks registered in the United States and other countries.

Printed in the U.S.A.

INTRODUCTION: HOW TO USE THIS BOOK

Finding A Test

This Encyclopedia describes over 650 different medical tests, listed in alphabetical order under the name most likely to be familiar to a patient. Many of these tests are known by a variety of names. For example, an ultrasound test, as it is most frequently designated, may also be called a Doppler test, sonography, sound scanning, or an echogram, depending on the doctor's specialty. The acid phosphatase test is often called the prostate test because of its specificity in revealing changes in that organ's activity. In some cases tests have been grouped according to function. For example, there are a great many thyroid tests using different techniques. But since all serve the same purpose—to measure the thyroid gland's activity—they are listed under a single heading: Thyroid Function. In all instances, the most common cross-reference terms are also listed alphabetically. If, for some reason, a particular test cannot be found, it may be known by another name.

New medical tests are, of course, being proposed, experimented with, and evaluated every day. At the same time, existing tests may become obsolete overnight as more efficient or convenient procedures are developed. It is impossible to include every medical test now available. Some tests are still without proven scientific value, and quite a few are limited to research investigations and are performed only in an academic hospital setting.

Each listing is accompanied by a brief description of what the test measures, when it is commonly performed, and the range of normal and abnormal values. For some tests, special problems or dangers are also noted.

Many tests are used to aid in the diagnosis of a large number of disease conditions. For example, the albumin/globulin test and certain enzyme determinations such as SGOT show changes in well over a hundred different illnesses. This Encyclopedia lists the most common conditions for which each test is performed.

Certain medical tests that may be used to aid in the diagnosis and treatment of some generalized medical conditions will be found in the Appendix: General Medical Conditions and Related Tests.

Interpreting A Test Value

The "normal" values cited for a test are those commonly accepted by the medical profession. Most laboratory test results are reported in numerical form. These values may vary with different laboratory procedures. For nonlaboratory tests such as X-rays, electrocardiograms, and reflex, or varicose vein observations, the doctor draws his own conclusions on the basis of his knowledge and experience. The normal values should be considered only as reference points. Some tests have such a wide range of values within normal limits that it takes a great deviation from the norm before any problem can be suspected.

To evaluate a test result, the patient need not understand the exact measure associated with a numerical value (for example, mg per 100 ml, mMol, mEq per L). The patient can simply compare the range of values considered normal—those found in 95 percent of healthy people—with his or her reported value.

Abnormal values are given numerically or descriptively, depending on the type of test. Again, only the most common conditions that cause abnormal test results are included. It cannot be emphasized enough that a single abnormal test value does not specifically signify a disease. The chances of error in medical testing are sufficiently great that any abnormal test must be repeated, preferably by a different physician or laboratory. When a reported abnormal test value is critical, most doctors will insist on a third trial before attributing significance to the results.

Patient-related causes of inaccurate test results

Many things a patient does in the course of daily activities can directly affect medical test results, causing them to have a false abnormal value.

Medications. Aspirin, laxatives, cold pills, cough preparations, sleeping aids, vitamins, nose drops, pain relievers, and especially stomach antacids can markedly alter a test value. Prescription drugs have an even greater influence on medical testing. In 1972 the American Association of Clinical Chemists published a list of over 9,000 different adverse effects on laboratory tests from drugs alone; the list has been growing ever since.

Birth control pills (oral conceptives), which many women do not regard as a medicine, can greatly alter the value of more than 60 medical tests, including 15 of those most frequently performed. Alcohol too can affect test values. A very small amount will distort blood pressure testing, lipid tests (such as cholesterol and triglycerides), the prothrombin time test, and any form of diabetes testing (glucose, insulin, etc.).

Before any test, the doctor or laboratory must be made aware of medications being used so that the medications can either be stopped before the test or be taken into account when the test results are evaluated.

Diet. A great many food substances can alter test results. For example, iodine from table salt, fish, hot dogs, or other foods can totally disrupt certain thyroid function tests. Foods containing large amounts of vitamin K (green leafy vegetables or fish) will cause prothrombin time tests to be abnormal. Some of the chemicals used in commercial French-fried potatoes will adversely affect the prothrombin time for a week. Drinking milk before a calcium or phosphorus test will lead to inaccurate results. Coffee can cause a false positive uric acid test. Even water can affect test results. There are times when water should be avoided prior to testing, just as there are times when a specified amount must be consumed. Taking bone meal tablets as a food supplement can cause cancer-like abnormalities on X-rays.

Routine activities. A patient's daily routine, including his sleeping habits, can have a direct effect on certain tests, especially hormone evaluations. If a patient works all night and sleeps during the day, the physician should be informed. Physical activity, or lack of it, can alter the results of a great many tests. For example, a renin test will have different results depending on whether a patient has been lying down or standing up just before the blood is taken.

Work-related factors must also be considered. Indirect contact with certain chemicals on the job can alter many test results. The amount of noise in a work location and even the lighting conditions can alter the body's hormone production, which in turn can change certain test results.

Attitude. If patients undergo stress or anxiety a few days before a test, or at the time the test is performed, the altered mental attitude can produce an abnormal test value. Patients who are kept waiting a long time for a test appointment may have false abnormal results. This is especially true if waiting causes the patient to miss another important appointment. Even having an attractive female technician take a blood sample from a male patient can alter test values.

Physical Factors. Sex, age, height, weight, and body surface area must be taken into account when interpreting the report of a medical test. It is perfectly normal for a woman to have a sedimentation rate twice as high as a man. Most pulmonary function tests and some hormone tests are dependent on size and physical build. Surprisingly, test results may vary in some people due to changes in the weather. Some families have genetic traits that give abnormal test values even though no true disease condition is present. More than 100 million people have an inherited glucose-6 phosphate dehydrogenase enzyme deficiency (rare in central European Caucasians), which causes a hemolytic type of anemia (destruction of red blood cells) in reaction to certain drugs and which would cause false abnormal test values for certain other types of anemia.

Technical Causes Of Abnormal Values

In addition to patient-related factors, technical problems in specimen collection and testing materials can lead to test inaccuracies. By being aware of these problems and minimizing them when possible, patients will be more likely to obtain accurate test results.

Specimen Collection. The taking of blood, usually from an arm vein, seems to be the most common cause of technically related laboratory test inaccuracies. Before inserting a needle for blood, the technician will usually tie a tourniquet (a piece of rubber tubing) tightly around the upper arm and then tell the patient to make a fist. If the tourniquet is left on for more than 30 seconds, or if the patient is asked to open and close the hand rapidly, an excessive amount of blood may accumulate in the arm below the tourniquet and abnormally high test values can result. To ensure accurate results in blood tests, the technician should apply the tourniquet to help locate a vein and then loosen it for at least 30 seconds before collecting the blood sample.

Most blood tests must be performed almost immediately after the blood is collected; a delay of only a few minutes can cause inaccurate test values. With patients taking anticoagulant drugs (to prevent blood clots), for example, a delay of more than ten minutes can markedly change the prothrombin time. As a result, the physician may prescribe a dangerously high (or low) dose of the anticoagulant.

If blood for a glucose test is left standing in a test tube for only one hour before it is tested, the glucose value can decrease by as much as 40 mg, or almost half of what is considered to be a normal value. The longer the tube of blood stands, the lower the glucose value. As a result, patients with diabetes may be wrongly told their sugar metabolism is perfectly normal.

Urine tests can also be affected by collection procedures. A "mid-stream, clean catch" is indicated for most urine tests. To ensure a clean specimen it is necessary to discard the first portion of the urine stream. Otherwise, the specimen may contain foreign material from the urethra (the passageway from the bladder to the outside), which can cause false abnormal values. Patients who are asked to collect a 24-hour urine specimen should use a special laboratory container with the proper preservative. The specimen should be kept under refrigeration during the collection period. If a preservative is not used, or if the urine specimen is allowed to stand at room temperature for more than an hour before testing, many of the test results will be incorrect.

Testing materials. Defects in test materials and equipment can also lead to erroneous test results. For example, the chemical reagent used in a test can cause inaccurate results if it is contaminated, mislabeled, or out of date. In its publication *Enforcement Report,* the Food and Drug Administration regularly reports on defective medical test reagents that have been seized by government officials or recalled by the manufacturer. Recently, some testing materials have been found to have incorrect or confusing instructions, again leading to false test values.

Many types of testing equipment (such as X-ray machines and electrocardiogram equipment) have virtually no standards to ensure accurate or uniform results. Their reliability depends on the skill of the technician and of the doctor who interprets the test results. The director of the FDA's Bureau of Radiological Health recently testified that 50,000 operators of X-ray machines meet no accreditation requirements and have no formal training in the equipment they use. Incorrect processing of X-ray pictures, even by trained X-ray technicians, can lead to misinterpretation of results and, ultimately, to erroneous diagnosis.

A recent survey of blood pressure gauges showed that one out of every four measuring devices gave erroneous readings—some showing such abnormally high blood pressure values that patients were unnecessarily treated for hypertension. It is an agreed-upon medical fact that multiple tests for blood pressure, at different times and under different circumstances, are essential in obtaining a true blood pressure reading. If the same defective instrument is used for each reading, a false abnormal value will be consistently reported. If the inflatable cuff wrapped around the upper arm is too small the blood pressure readings will be elevated.

The Risk Factors In Medical Testing

In medical testing, as in all facets of medicine, including drug therapy and surgery, the risks must be weighed against the expected benefits. One of the greatest hazards in testing is excessive exposure to X-rays, which can cause damage to the body such as hair loss and cancer.

Another hazard in medical testing involves invasion of body tissues. Whenever a catheter (thin tube) is inserted into a blood vessel to inject a dye or other substance into the body, the patient runs the risk of infection, trauma, or allergic reaction. At the present time one out of every 40,000 patients has a fatal reaction to radiography of the kidney, after a dye is injected to outline the urinary tract. With nuclear scanning tests, in which radioactive chemicals are injected into the body, one out of every 1,000 patients has an adverse reaction.

With today's technology, the hazards posed by injecting a needle into an arm vein are quite remote. Still, the patient runs some risk of infection or of extravasation (the blood seeps out into the tissues of the arm under the skin, causing nerve, muscle, and skin damage). When medical tests are performed with electrical instruments, burns and even fatal shocks can result if the machines have not been properly grounded or maintained.

The risk involved in medical testing must always be weighed against the potential benefits to the patient. No test procedure should be viewed as harmless, especially if it involves invasion of body tissues. On the other hand, a medical test can be life-saving to a patient, helping the physician diagnose a condition at an early stage, when cure is possible.

Finally, it must be stressed that this book is not a manual for self-diagnosis. Although some tests may be indicative of specific disease processes, no test, or even battery of tests, can be considered conclusive in determining the cause, the presence, or the absence of illness. Even when an abnormal test value is consistent, it alone may not be considered diagnostic. A medical test must always be interpreted in the context of the patient's symptoms and the doctor's other findings. A test in itself is relatively meaningless; it is only one of many guides to a patient's health.

AAT, see *Albumin/Globulin*

ABDOMINAL ENDOSCOPY, see *Endoscopy*

ABORTION WARNING, see *Placental Lactogen*

ABSCESS CULTURE, see *Culture*

ACCOMMODATION, see *Visual Acuity*

ACETYLCHOLINESTERASE, see *Cholinesterase*

ACG, see *Apexcardiogram*

ACHILLES REFLEX, see *Thyroid Function*

ACID-BASE BALANCE, see *pH*

ACID-FAST STAIN, see *Culture*

ACID HEMOLYSIS, see *HAM*

ACIDOSIS, see *Carbon Dioxide*; *Ketones*; *pH*

ACID PHOSPHATASE

Acid phosphatase is an enzyme found primarily in the prostate gland. The male hormone testosterone causes the prostate to secrete acid phosphatase into the bloodstream. Blood is taken from an arm vein for serum examination. Urine and prostatic secretion are occasionally tested. Direct aspiration of the prostate by needle is also used to test for prostate disease.

When performed: If there is a suspected abnormality of the prostate gland; to help identify metastasizing carcinomas (spreading cancers).

In suspected rape the vaginal fluid may be tested for prostatic acid phosphatase to prove sexual intercourse took place. Many rapists have abnormal sex gland functioning and do not produce sperm; a woman who has been raped may not show a positive sperm test but will usually show a positive acid phosphatase test. In addition, sperm may disappear after a day or two, but the acid phosphatase will remain for at least 72 hours.

Normal values: Several different methods are used to measure acid phosphatase; the values vary with the method used. The most common values are 0 to 2.0 Bodansky units; 0 to 0.65 Bessey-Lowry units; 0 to 5.0 King-Armstrong units; and 1 to 1.9 IU per liter.

Abnormal values: Acid phosphatase is elevated with metastatic carcinoma (spreading cancer) of the prostate and the spread of some other cancers (a normal acid phosphatase is not an assurance of no cancer), Paget's disease (thickening and softening of the bones), and a form of bone cancer called multiple myeloma. The King-Armstrong method can detect moderate rises in cases of pneumonia, hepatitis, as well as with certain cancers. The Bodansky method is more specific for prostatic cancer. Prostatic examination or massage will also elevate serum acid phosphatase levels, as will the taking of the drug clofibrate (Atromid-S).

Note: The newer radioimmunoassay technique to detect acid phosphatase is of such increased sensitivity, it may allow even earlier diagnosis of prostate cancer.

ACROMEGALY, see *Growth Hormone*

ACTH STIMULATION, see *Cortisol*

ACTIVATED PARTIAL THROMBOPLASTIN TIME, see *Partial Thromboplastin Time*

ADDIS COUNT, see *Urine Examination*

ADRENAL CORTICAL, see *Cortisol*

ADRENALIN, see *Catecholamines*

ADRENALIN MEDULLA, see *Catecholamines*

ADRENAL SUPPRESSION, see *Cortisol*

AFP, see *Alpha Fetoprotein*

AGGLUTINATION

Agglutination means the clumping or gathering together of cells (usually red blood cells) into a mass instead of each cell existing separately. This phenomenon can easily be seen under the microscope; in many instances it can also be viewed with the naked eye when the lumps settle into the bottom of a test tube or clump together on a glass slide.

Agglutination occurs as a reaction against various diseases, primarily infections. Whenever the body is exposed to bacteria, viruses, fungus, or a toxin that contains antigens (the agents that cause disease), it reacts by producing antibodies. These antibodies then attempt to fight off the specific organism invasion. Antibodies found in a patient's blood indicate that the patient has already been exposed to a particular infection. The exposure may have occurred many years previously or it may be of very recent origin.

The principle behind agglutination testing is always the same: to see if antigens of a known condition have already caused a defensive (antibody) reaction against that condition. If antibodies are present and clump with the known antigen, the test is called positive. Some antigens combine with antibodies only in cold temperatures, some need warm temperatures, some clump better when exposed to latex particles, and some show clumping best when sheep red blood cells previously exposed to the disease are used. Sometimes the cells flocculate, or fall like snowflakes, clumping at the bottom of the tube.

A single positive agglutination test is not usually sufficient to make a diagnosis. To determine if the disease is recent enough to be the cause of a patient's symptoms, two or three agglutination tests are performed within a few weeks. The serum is diluted first with equal parts of an innocuous solution and then progressively down to one part serum to well over a thousand parts of diluent (e.g., 1:1,064). The result is reported by titer (the highest titer represents the weakest solution in which agglutination occurs). A noticeable rise in titer with each test usually indicates an active disease with more and more antibodies being formed daily. Blood is taken from a vein and the serum is tested. Thus sometimes the test is called "serology."

A related test, **Complement Fixation,** is also used to diagnose mysterious infections. The two tests may be given together. At times the same disease will give a positive reaction to the agglutination test as well as the complement fixation test. At other times a particular disease will respond only to one of them.

Coombs' test for agglutination (there is a Direct Coombs' and an Indirect Coombs') is used primarily in blood conditions. A positive Direct Coombs' usually signifies erythroblastosis fetalis (the Rh anemia of newborns) and hemolytic anemia (where a person's own antibodies destroy his red blood cells). The Indirect Coombs' is used to detect Rh blood-type factors. Unfortunately, a great many drugs, including penicillin, cause a positive Direct Coombs'.

When performed: The test is used most often when there is a persistent fever, such as occurs with an infection that cannot be diagnosed. Specific infections for which different forms of agglutination tests are conducted include:

Amebiasis

Brucellosis
> (undulant fever, usually resulting from association with cows, sheep, or goats and their unpasteurized milk)

American trypanosomiasis
> (a form of sleeping sickness)

Cryptococcosis
> (a fungus-caused meningitis)

German measles or Rubella
> (an agglutination test is required by law in some states at time of

marriage or pregnancy to see if a prospective mother has ever had the disease and to immunize her if she never did)

Histoplasmosis
   (a fungus-caused lung infection)
Infectious mononucleosis
Leptospirosis
   (hemmorhagic jaundice)
Measles
Melioidosis
   (generalized infection common in drug addicts)
Mumps
Q-fever
   (a rickettsial pneumonia; rickettsia are a form of bacteria)
Rat-bite fever
Schistosomiasis
   (swimmer's itch)
Streptococcal infections
Toxoplasmosis
   (muscle infection, primarily from touching cat feces; especially dangerous in pregnancy)
Trichinosis
   (mostly from eating raw, infected pork)
Tularemia
   (rabbit-handling fever)
Typhoid fever
Typhus
Viral pneumonia

Agglutination tests are also performed to help diagnose rheumatoid arthritis; to ascertain the specific cause of certain allergic reactions such as to cow's milk; to diagnose certain anemias caused by the Rh factor; to determine a person's blood type such as A, B, AB, O, or Rh; and even to ascertain pregnancy.

By noting which type of blood a person's serum agglutinates, the physician can determine that person's blood type and therefore the type of blood that would be safe for transfusion if ever needed. Whether a mother will react to the Rh factor during pregnancy is also determined in the same way. By mixing a woman's urine that contains the hormone increased during pregnancy with the antiserum for that hormone and observing for agglutination, the physician can ascertain if the woman is pregnant.

Normal values: While agglutination reactions to disease should not be present, an old, forgotten infection can cause a positive test. Usually, though, the titer is quite low, averaging less than a 1:64 dilution. Unless this titer suddenly rises (is present in much greater dilutions) within a few days, it is not considered evidence of any active disease. When it comes to blood typing, there are no normal values.

Abnormal values: If the titer of a patient against a specific disease rises within a few days to a week, it can reasonably be concluded that the patient is manufacturing a great many antibodies against that disease and therefore is harboring the organism that causes the disease. Sometimes agglutination tests are performed against a number of different infectious diseases; the one that shows the highest, increasing titer usually indicates the diagnosis. A titer over 1:64 is needed to be of definitive value.

Well over half of all people with rheumatoid arthritis show a positive agglutination test to latex particles (the reason is not known), but then so do some people with systemic lupus erythematosus and chronic infections. A few drugs such as methyldopa (for high blood pressure) and some pain relievers can cause a false positive test; in contrast, excessive use of certain antibiotics can mask a positive agglutination test, making it appear negative.

AGGREGOMETER, see *Platelet Count*

A/G RATIO, see *Albumin/Globulin*

ALA, see *Lead*; *Porphyrins*

ALANINE AMINOTRANSFERASE (ALT), see *Glutamic Oxalacetic Transaminase*

ALBUMIN/GLOBULIN (A/G Ratio)

Albumin and globulins are the main total plasma proteins in the blood. These proteins aid in maintaining the osmotic pressure of the blood (keeping a balance between the percentage of chemicals and plasma), provide nutritive substance for tissues, and carry essential substances such as hormones, vitamins, drugs, and enzymes throughout the body. There are four different globulins; the largest in number are the gamma globulins, which carry the immune bodies to help fight disease. The average person produces about 15 g of plasma proteins a day. Blood is taken from a vein and the plasma or serum is tested. The results are stated as a ratio of the amount of albumin to the amount of all the globulins.

Albumin and globulin are also measured in other body fluids; the presence of albumin (protein) in the urine is an indicator of kidney disease. However, people with a condition known as orthostatic albuminuria automatically excrete albumin in the urine when they are on their feet for long periods of time. It signifies no disease.

When performed: If there are problems of food absorption; to distinguish starvation from other diseases; in various liver and kidney diseases; when there is a question of infections, especially when there seems to be no resistance to infection.

Normal values: The total proteins (primarily the sum of the albumin and the globulins) average 7 g per 100 ml. Usually there is almost twice as much albumin, 4.5 g per 100 ml, as there are globulins, 2.5 g per 100 ml; and when the amount of albumin is divided by the amount of globulins, the normal A/G ratio averages two to one (2:1). Ratios from 1.5:1 to 2.5:1 are within normal limits.

Abnormal values: With diseases that affect the blood proteins, the amount of albumin is usually decreased and the globulins increased, thereby reversing the usual A/G ratio. In liver conditions especially, the amount of albumin decreases because of that organ's inability to manufacture it; gamma globulins increase, since they are made outside the liver. In kidney problems both the serum albumin and gamma globulins decrease, but the alpha and beta globulins increase. In starvation, because little or no protein is eaten, all the blood proteins are decreased. The same decrease in the proteins is found when food cannot be absorbed because of various diseases.

Alpha antitrypsin (AAT), an antienzyme globulin, is decreased in inherited liver disease in children and lung disease in adults. Another globulin, **Alpha Fetoprotein** (AFP), usually disappears from the blood after birth but is sometimes found in adults with liver and other cancers.

ALCOHOL

Testing for the body's ethyl alcohol content—whether in the blood, the breath, or the urine—is most commonly related to the legal question of driving while drunk. Police and highway officers often measure alcohol concentration in the breath, which reflects blood levels. After alcohol is consumed, it reaches a peak in the blood in about half an hour's time. It takes about three hours to eliminate each ounce of alcohol ingested. Thus a blood alcohol test is fairly reliable for many hours after the last drink. The blood alcohol test is also an important diagnostic tool when an unconscious person is brought to an emergency facility.

Blood, breath, or urine may be tested. Blood is taken from a vein. Breath is usually collected in a bag or balloon, or it may be exhaled directly into a measuring instrument. In the urine test, the individual must first empty the bladder and then wait a minimum of 20 minutes before the test sample is taken so that the specimen accurately reflects the amount of body alcohol at the time of testing.

When performed: The test is performed not only to determine if alcohol has been consumed but, of greater importance, to determine the degree of alcoholic intoxication so as to apply proper treatment. It can also help determine the cause of coma and is used to discriminate antihistamine or tranquilizer overdosage from alcohol toxicity.

Normal values: Normally there is no measurable amount of alcohol in the body. When less than 0.05% of the blood (50 mg per 100 ml) is composed of alcohol, it is usually not considered intoxication in the legal sense.

Abnormal values: Three ounces of an average (86-proof) liquor will usually produce symptoms of intoxication and cause a blood alcohol level of over 0.05%, which in many states is sufficient to cause prosecution as "under the influence." Other states have laws that stipulate more than 0.10% as evidence of intoxication; a few states insist on alcohol levels of 0.15% before issuing a citation. Ten ounces of liquor will usually produce stupor or coma and will cause blood alcohol levels to measure 0.4%. Twelve ounces at one time has caused death. Urine levels are always about 50% higher than corresponding blood levels. Breath values parallel blood values.

Abnormally high test values will result if, just prior to inserting the needle to take blood, the technician wipes the skin with alcohol, or if the individual belches while breathing into a bag or measuring device. The use of alcohol-containing mouthwashes prior to a breathing test can also cause higher values.

ALCOHOLISM

The **Alcohol** test (whether from blood, breath, or urine) is a measure of the amount of alcohol in a person at the time the test is taken. It does not in any way indicate whether the patient is a chronic user of alcohol. There are, however, tests that can reveal whether a person is a heavy drinker, or even an alcoholic, in spite of that person's denial. One such test is the measurement of enzymes, either gamma glutamyl transferase (GGT) or gamma glutamyl transpeptidase (GGTP). Others include the folic acid test (see **Folates**), **Uric Acid** test, measurement of **Zinc** levels in the blood or urine, measurement of **Sweat**, and measurement of certain amino acids in the blood such as alpha-amino-n-butyric acid and glutamate dehydrogenase (GDH) that indicate liver damage.

When performed: Whenever alcoholism is suspected or when patients are admitted to hospitals in coma or undiagnosed unconscious conditions; to aid in uncovering patients who might become alcoholics; to aid in the treatment of patients who show symptoms of alcoholism but who deny drinking; to follow the progress of a patient's therapy.

Normal values: Normal values range from 30 to 45 units per liter (men usually have higher amounts) for GGT; less than 25 units per liter for GGTP. Amino acids have varying normal values.

Abnormal values: GGT will rise to 500 to 1,000 units per liter depending on how heavily the person has been drinking and for how long; the GGTP enzyme will usually go above 250 units per liter. Normal amino acids will double in alcoholics. Folic acid will decrease, and uric acid will increase. It takes more than 5 ounces of alcohol a day, on a regular basis, to affect these test values; but the greater the alcohol intake, the higher the test value.

ALDOLASE

Aldolase is an enzyme that helps convert sugar in the muscles to energy. Like another enzyme, **Lactic Dehydrogenase** (LDH), aldolase is found in increased quantities in the blood when there is severe damage to various body tissues, especially muscles. In addition to its concentration in skeletal muscle tissue, aldolase is found in the liver, heart muscle, and red blood cells. Blood is withdrawn from a vein and the serum is examined.

When performed: Aldolase measurement is used mainly in muscle disorders, particularly in early diagnosis of spinal muscle atrophy conditions.

Normal values: Values vary with the method used. A range of 0 to 12 units per ml is considered normal.

Abnormal values: Aldolase is increased in the blood primarily with polymyositis (infected muscles), muscular dystrophy, acute hepatitis, infectious mononucleosis, crush injury, malignancies (especially liver and prostate), various anemias, heart attack, pulmonary embolism, delirium tremens, stroke, trichinosis, pneumonia, hemorrhagic pancreatitis, and lead intoxication.

ALDOSTERONE

Aldosterone is a hormone of the adrenal gland that controls the electrolyte balance (see **Chloride**; **Potassium**; **Sodium**) in the body. (Other adrenal hormone groups are the cortisones and the adrenalins.) By keeping sodium (which holds fluid) in and letting potassium out of the body, aldosterone controls the volume of the blood and therefore, in part, blood pressure. Normally, the amount of aldosterone in the body is regulated by **Renin**, an enzyme produced by the kidney; renin, in turn, reacts to blood sodium changes and blood volume. Renin is sometimes measured alone, usually when blood pressure problems are thought to be caused by only one kidney; more often it is measured with aldosterone as a means of diagnosing where an aldosterone-forming tumor is located. Blood is taken from a vein and the plasma is tested. Urine is also measured for aldosterone.

When performed: With high blood pressure; when an adrenal tumor is suspected; when there is a constant problem with sodium and/or potassium control; when there is edema (water retention) that cannot be explained.

Normal values: Plasma levels should not exceed 20 ng per 100 ml. Urine levels should be no more than 20 ng per 24-hour specimen. Normal values from various laboratories may differ markedly.

Abnormal values: Elevated aldosterone values (usually along with decreased potassium and increased sodium) indicate hyperaldosteronism, which can come from an adrenal tumor, kidney disease, or liver disease. Elevated levels may also occur following surgery and during pregnancy. Sometimes a salt-loading test is performed: after several days on a salt-free diet, the patient is given a large amount of sodium; normally this stops production of aldosterone, and the salt is passed out in the urine. With aldosterone problems, the patient's body retains the sodium and becomes edematous.

ALKALINE PHOSPHATASE

Alkaline phosphatase is an enzyme normally found in the blood. Different forms of this enzyme are also produced in the intestines, liver, and bone cells. Conditions that stimulate bone cell activity and that deposit excess calcium in the bones create elevated alkaline phosphatase levels in the blood. A single test for alkaline phosphatase is insufficient for diagnosis; it must be evaluated several times. Blood is usually taken from an arm vein for serum examination. All urine passed in an 8-hour period (usually overnight) may also be tested. In certain rare diseases alkaline phosphatase is also observed in white blood cells.

When performed: When cancer is suspected; to differentiate the causes of liver disease; following injury; when parathyroid disease is suspected; to study nutritional problems such as **Vitamin D** deficiency.

Normal values: Values vary with the kind of test measurement used: 2 to 4.5 Bodansky units; 0.8 to 2.3 Bessey-Lowry units; 3.0 to 13.0 King-Armstrong units. Normal values are higher in children because of bone growth activity.

Abnormal values: Higher than normal values are found with cancerous and noncancerous bone disease, liver disease, blockage of the bile duct system (gall bladder disease), Gaucher's disease (a type of anemia), healing fractures, rickets, leukemia, thyroid gland infection, and hyperparathyroidism; values may also rise during the latter part of pregnancy. Elevated alkaline phosphatase levels are caused by a number of drugs, including male hormones, tranquilizers such as Thorazine, antibiotics such as erythromycin and oxacillin, some antiarthritic drugs such as gold and Indocin, and oral antidiabetic drugs. Birth control pills will also elevate alkaline phosphatase levels.

Lower than normal values are found in patients taking too much vitamin D or too little vitamin C, and in conditions of poor nutrition. Patients taking Atromid-S to reduce blood cholesterol levels have been reported to have falsely lowered alkaline phosphatase levels, which could mask the diagnosis of certain liver diseases; it has also been noted that patients who take Atromid-S have a much greater incidence of gall bladder disease.

ALKALOSIS, see *Carbon Dioxide*; *pH*

ALKAPTONURIA, see *Aminoaciduria*

ALLERGY, see *RAST*; *Skin Reaction*

ALPHA-AMINO-N-BUTYRIC ACID, see *Alcoholism*

ALPHA ANTITRYPSIN, see *Albumin/Globulin*

ALPHA CHOLESTEROL, see *Cholesterol*

ALPHA FETOPROTEIN

Alpha fetoprotein is the primary serum protein (see **Albumin/Globulin**) of the fetus during pregnancy; it usually disappears totally from the newborn's blood immediately after birth. Should it reappear in later life, it most likely indicates liver cell pathology. Blood is taken from a vein and the serum is tested. Amniotic fluid (the fluid around the fetus) is also tested.

When performed: When liver disease, especially liver cell cancer, is suspected; when a cancer (most likely from the ovary or testicle) is thought to have spread to the liver; as a means of following the progress of therapy in the treatment of hepatitis.

Normal values: Normally no alpha fetoprotein is found in the blood except in pregnancy. During pregnancy up to 2.5 mg per 100 ml may be detected in the amniotic fluid, depending on the month of gestation.

Abnormal values: Any amount found in the blood serum of an adult (young children may still have a trace) is abnormal and commonly indicates a liver cell cancer; however, it can on occasion be found in other cancers and thus is not an absolute diagnostic indicator. It sometimes appears during recovery from hepatitis. When **alpha fetoprotein** is increased in amniotic fluid, it can indicate a problem with the fetus.

ALPHA HYDROXYBUTYRIC DEHYDROGENASE, see *Hydroxybutyric Dehydrogenase*

ALPHA-2 MACROGLOBULIN, see *Macroglobulin*

ALPHA TOCOPHEROL, see *Tocopherols*

ALPHA WAVE, see *Electroencephalogram*

ALT, see *Glutamic Oxalacetic Transaminase*

AMBLYOPIA, see *Visual Acuity*

AMEBIASIS, see *Agglutination*

AMETROPIA, see *Visual Acuity*

AMINOACIDURIA

Abnormal amounts of amino acids appear in the urine whenever there are certain inborn (inherited) errors of metabolism. There are nearly 2,000 known inherited diseases of this type (see, for example, **Phenylketonuria**), but only about two dozen have regular test procedures. There are also a few similar conditions that are acquired after birth. Each condition has some unique way of manifesting itself. For example, cystinuria causes kidney stones; alkaptonuria causes a form of arthritis; Hartnup's disease is primarily a skin condition; maple syrup urine disease (so named because the urine takes on a maple syrup odor) can cause convulsions; and homocystinuria can bring about eye problems.

In most instances, because of the missing enzyme, the kidney cannot handle the faulty metabolism of certain amino acids from proteins that are eaten. There is also a degree of mental retardation in many of these difficulties. Urine and plasma may be screened for general amino acid abnormalities, but in most instances tests for specific amino acid excess are performed on the basis of the patient's symptoms.

When performed: Most often on newborn infants, but also on young children (occasionally on adults with appropriate symptoms) who show signs of retardation or other inherited abnormalities.

Normal values: Each of the 29 amino acids and their metabolites has a different normal value. In the blood the levels are usually high at birth and lessen with age. In the urine the opposite is the rule.

Abnormal values: Increased amounts in the plasma and urine not only help diagnose the condition but can also indicate specific dietary treatment, which is usually successful.

AMMONIA

Ammonia is usually produced in the liver, intestines, and kidneys as an end product of protein metabolism. The liver converts ammonia into urea to be excreted by the kidneys. In liver disease the conversion of ammonia to urea is diminished, producing an increase in blood ammonia levels. Whole blood from a vein is examined. Ammonia may be measured in the urine by taking a sample of all urine passed during a 24-hour period.

When performed: If there is suspicion of liver disease or other conditions that affect liver function.

Normal values: Values vary with different laboratories, but generally 75 mcg per 100 ml of blood is considered normal. The urine usually contains up to 1 g in a 24-hour sample.

Abnormal values: Blood ammonia is increased in liver disease, especially in portal system encephalopathy or abnormal mental states due to poor liver function. It may also be elevated when patients are taking diuretics (thiazides, Diamox) and antibiotics (methicillin) or when there is an increase in certain amino acids (from proteins) in the blood, usually an inherited condition.

AMNIOCENTESIS

Studying the amniotic fluid (the fluid that surrounds the fetus during pregnancy) is becoming commonplace when it is suspected that a child might be born with an inherited defect. In the United States more than 100,000 children are born each year with some form of developmental disability. The fetus gives off cells while growing, and these cells can be studied directly. The test is usually performed early in pregnancy (after 15 weeks), but it can also be done before delivery to insure that the fetus is sufficiently mature to survive.

After locating the exact position of the fetus, usually with the **Ultrasound** test, the physician places a long thin needle through the abdomen into the uterus and withdraws the fluid. There is a risk of one out of every 200 children being aborted by the test. The test can usually determine the sex of the fetus, but many people do not wish to know this fact before birth. Sex determination is not 100% accurate, however; errors occur in about one out of every 20 tests.

Many different metabolic conditions can be diagnosed prior to birth (Down's syndrome, Tay-Sachs disease, some malformations). The process is called karyotyping (chromosome analysis), or comparing the fetal chromosome size, shape, and number to what is known to be normal, thus predicting the genetic status of the unborn infant. Chromosome analysis is also performed from blood samples on young children and adults when there are sex identification problems or a question of an inherited abnormality. The same type of test can be performed on blood cells and other body tissues. (The Tay-Sachs blood-screening test for potential parents can help determine the probability of having children with Tay-Sachs disease.)

Amniotic fluid is also tested for **Alpha fetoprotein** and **Bilirubin**.

When performed: The test is especially applicable to pregnant women over 35 years of age; families who have relatives with metabolic problems; families who have children born with Down's syndrome; and families who have past indications of chromosome abnormalities. It is also used when there have been cases of mental retardation in the family; when there is a question of an Rh problem; to offer genetic counseling early enough in pregnancy; to determine the sex and maturity of the unborn child; and to diagnose the "funny-looking kid" syndrome.

Normal values: Chromosomal analysis shows no defect.

Abnormal values: When chromosomal patterns show either excessive or missing genes; when certain genes are translocated or found on the wrong chromosomes; when chromosomes are broken. More than 80 different metabolic diseases may now be diagnosed through chromosome analysis and additional congenital abnormalities continue to be discovered yearly.

An excess of alpha fetoprotein in amniotic fluid usually indicates a neurological defect; the degree of increase in bilirubin helps predict how serious an Rh baby's condition will be after birth.

AMYLASE

Amylase (composed of several enzymes used in the digestion of starch) is normally found in very small amounts in blood serum. It is produced in the pancreas, the salivary glands, the fallopian tubes, and mostly in the liver. Blood is drawn from an arm vein and the serum is examined. The urine is also tested.

When performed: When abdominal pain suggests pancreatitis; for mumps, pancreas duct obstruction, acute renal (kidney) insufficiency, and intestinal obstruction.

Normal values: Normal serum levels range from 80 to 150 Somogyi units per 100 ml. Normal urine shows from 1,000 to 5,000 Somogyi units per 24-hour sample.

Abnormal values: Amylase levels are increased primarily with pancreatitis, pancreas duct obstruction, salivary gland or duct problems (mumps), perforated ulcer, intestinal obstruction, and renal insufficiency. Amylase levels may also be elevated by certain drugs, including codeine, a large amount of alcohol, indomethacin (Indocin), meperidine (Demerol), morphine, pentazocine (Talwin), and thiazide diuretics. An elevated amylase level becomes even more specific for pancreatitis if the urine shows an increase in amylase clearance by the kidneys when compared with **Creatinine** clearance. Amylase levels may be lower than normal in hepatitis or liver damage or when there is trauma to or deficient functioning of the pancreas so that it is unable to produce the enzyme.

ANA, see *Antinuclear Antibodies*

ANGIOGRAPHY, see *Radiography*

ANGIOTENSIN, see *Renin*

ANION GAP, see *Lactic Acid*

ANISOMETROPIA, see *Visual Acuity*

ANTIBIOTIC SENSITIVITY, see *Culture*

ANTIBODY, see *Immunoglobulin*

ANTICOAGULANT, see *Prothrombin Time*

ANTICONVULSANT DRUG, see *Drug Monitoring*

ANTIFREEZE, see *Methanol*

ANTINUCLEAR ANTIBODIES (ANA)

Antigens such as bacteria, toxins, tissue cells, or foreign proteins are provocative factors in many illnesses. They induce the body to produce antibodies to fight the antigens. The antibodies attempt to combine with the antigens in order to neutralize them. In certain rare and unique diseases, the body's immune system, whose main function is to resist disease, produces antibodies to parts of the patient's own body. These antibodies are special forms of gamma globulins called immunoglobulins and seem to affect all parts of the body that have nucleoprotein, especially muscles and skin. They are called antinuclear antibodies and are found most commonly in people with systemic lupus erythematosus (SLE); they may also be found in people who have relatives suffering from SLE but who do not themselves have the disease.

Blood is taken from a vein and the serum is examined under the microscope after a fluorescent dye is added. Antinuclear antibodies will appear to fluoresce if they are present. When the ANA test is positive, the serum is then diluted, first in half, then in a 1:4 dilution, a 1:8 dilution, a 1:16 dilution, and so on. The weaker the dilution that fluoresces, the more positive the test.

The lupus erythematosus (LE) cell test is a form of ANA test that is sometimes more specific for SLE. It is considered "positive" when an antinuclear antibody combines with white blood cells and offers a characteristic LE cell picture (grouping) when viewed under the microscope. Several LE cells must be seen to constitute a positive test. Eighty percent of people with SLE have positive LE cell tests.

When performed: The ANA test is used primarily when there is suspicion of systemic lupus erythematosus (SLE). It is also performed when a patient has a variety of unexplained symptoms such as mysterious rash, arthritis, or chest pains that cannot easily be diagnosed.

Normal values: Antinuclear antibodies are not usually found in the blood. Their presence, though, does not always mean disease, as when found in close relatives of people with SLE.

Abnormal values: Abnormal levels are found mostly with SLE, which usually produces the highest titers (the presence of ANA in the weakest dilutions of serum); scleroderma (marked thickening of the skin) and rheumatoid arthritis usually cause ANA to be observed but in much lower titers (very little dilution). Some forms of kidney disease and certain infections of the pleura (lining around the lungs) can cause ANA. Many drugs can cause a false positive test: certain thiazide diuretics, almost all antibiotics (penicillin, Terramycin, isoniazid), some tranquilizers such as Taractin, the oral contraceptive pills, a few drugs used to treat high blood pressure (Apresoline), and procainamide, which is used primarily to treat heartbeat irregularities, but is sometimes used as an unproven youth restorer. The presence of ANA may be masked or hidden (false negative) even with disease if the patient is taking steroid drugs.

ANTISTREPTOLYSIN O (ASO) TITER

Streptococcal infection such as sore throat causes production of a number of antibodies (the body's defense reaction) that can be detected in the blood. One of these is antistreptolysin O. Blood from a vein is withdrawn and the serum is examined.

When performed: The test is used primarily when rheumatic fever or kidney disease (glomerulonephritis) is suspected as a complication of recent streptococcal infection. A single antibody test is usually insufficient to establish a recent infection. Several serial tests are necessary to show the sudden rise in the antibodies.

Normal values: Normally antistreptolysin O antibodies are not present, or if present are found in negligible amounts, usually under 150 Todd units per ml.

Abnormal values: ASO is elevated after a recent streptococcal infection. More than 175 Todd units per ml is indicative of such infection, but of even greater importance is an increasing value over several days' time. High readings have also been found in hepatitis, biliary obstruction, and nephrosis.

ANTITHYROID ANTIBODY, see *Thyroid Function*

APEXCARDIOGRAM (ACG)

An apexcardiogram (ACG) is a variation of the standard **Electrocardiogram** (ECG). In the apexcardiogram a transducer (an electrical device that detects pressure, vibrations, and temperature and translates that energy into recordable tracings to be viewed) is applied to the chest just above the heart. (The apex of the heart is the point that is usually lowest and farthest to the left—what might graphically be described as the "point" of the heart's shape.)

In essence, the apexcardiograph picks up and records the same heart contraction vibrations that can sometimes be seen on the surface of the chest and that can be felt when a hand is applied to the area. The ACG is considered noninvasive, since it is an external technique and the heart itself is not touched directly. An apexcardiogram is rarely ever performed without an accompanying **Phonocardiogram** (the same instrument is used to perform this test) and an **Electrocardiogram** (ECG).

A somewhat analogous form of apexcardiography is called kinetocardiography. This test, which some say is a bit more sensitive, requires a much more complicated apparatus. The kinetocardiograph records from a fixed point above a patient's chest (not directly touching the body), while the apexcardiograph can be directed specifically to the heart's apex.

When performed: To graphically identify the vibrations made by heart sounds, especially when abnormal ones are suspected; to verify heart valve disease; to detect tumors of the heart muscle.

Normal values: As with the ECG, the rises and falls of the lines (waves) produced by the instrument are translated into normalcy, suspicion of, or indication of disease by virtue of the experience of the physician interpreting the waves. Patients who are quite fat or who have large, barrel chests from emphysema may not produce sufficient waves for interpretation.

Abnormal values: The recordings show abnormalities in the way the blood travels through the heart; when there is disease, various notches and interruptions in the normally smooth, consistent recorded lines (waves) are evident. Heart valve problems are particularly detectable by this technique, as are abnormal pressure changes within the heart's chambers.

APHAKIA, see *Visual Acuity*

APHASIA, see *Language Function*

APPLANATION, see *Tonometry*

ARGENTAFFINOMA, see *Serotonin*

ARGYLL-ROBERTSON, see *Pupillary Reflex*

ARMY GENERAL CLASSIFICATION, see *Intelligence Quotient*

ART, see *Syphilis*

ARTHRITIS, see *Synovial Fluid*

ARTHROCENTESIS, see *Synovial Fluid*

ARTHROGRAPHY, see *Radiography*

ASCORBIC ACID (Vitamin C)

Because of a genetically transmitted defect, the human is one of very few mammals that cannot manufacture its own vitamin C. Although ascorbic acid is not stored in large amounts in the body, it is still essential to the body's defense mechanisms (resistance to all forms of disease) and to the formation of bones and teeth. While scurvy (severe vitamin C deficiency disease) is relatively uncommon, slight deficiencies do exist today. Anemia may occur in infants with vitamin C deficiency. Cancer patients often have low blood ascorbic acid levels even with an adequate diet and vitamin supplements. Blood is collected from a vein and the plasma is examined. Urinary ascorbic acid may also be examined.

When performed: In patients who present scurvylike symptoms (fatigue, loss of appetite, small hemorrhages under the skin and in the gums, hair problems); in patients with severe burns, infections, or malignancies.

Normal values: Normal values range from 0.6 to 2.0 mg per 100 ml of plasma, reflecting the 5 g of vitamin C normally found in the body; 20 mg of ascorbic acid is usually excreted daily in the urine.

Abnormal values: Lower than normal values are found with scurvy, cancer, severe infections, and alcoholism. Vitamin C deficiency is also found in infants fed only milk and in patients with hiatal hernia.

ASO, see *Antistreptolysin O Titer*

Aspartate Aminotransferase (AST), see *Glutamic Oxalacetic Transaminase*

ASPERGILLOSIS, see *Complement Fixation*

ASPIRIN, see *Salicylates*

ASPIRIN ALLERGY, see *Tartrazine Sensitivity*

AST, see *Glutamic Oxalacetic Transaminase*

ASTIGMATISM, see *Visual Acuity*

ATA, see *Thyroid Function*

ATYPICAL LYMPHOCYTE, see *Mononucleosis*

AUDIOMETER, see *Hearing Function*

AUSTRALIAN ANTIGEN (AU)

The Australian antigen (AU) test is also called the hepatitis B surface antigen (HBsAg) test, the hepatitis-associated antigen (HAA) test, the serum hepatitis (SH) test, and the hepatitis B (HB) test. The test, which was first performed successfully on an Australian aborigine (hence its name) in 1964, distinguishes between the two best-known types of virus-caused infectious hepatitis. Type A, the most common (usually called infectious hepatitis), is caused primarily by eating food containing the virus or by being in close contact with someone who has, or recently had, the disease. Type B is called serum hepatitis and is almost always transmitted when a needle or other instrument contaminated with the virus breaks the skin (such as when receiving an injection or intravenous solutions or during surgery). Type B is a much more serious illness, causing ten times as many deaths as type A.

There are several other varieties of the Australian antigen, one of which is more specific in drug addicts. A Type C virus was recently isolated. Blood is taken from a vein and the serum examined. The test is usually repeated a few days later for confirmation.

When performed: Primarily to distinguish type B from type A hepatitis (type A will usually respond to gamma globulin injections); to distinguish hepatitis from somewhat similar diseases such as infectious mononucleosis and other virus infections; to test all blood donated for transfusions.

Normal values: Normally no AU is detectable in the blood. It is, however, routinely found in a very small number of Americans who have no symptoms and in a large percentage of people who live in Asia and the Middle East. Those with type A hepatitis do not have a positive AU test.

Abnormal values: AU is positive in individuals who have become infected with type B hepatitis virus; it can become positive up to two weeks before a patient has any symptoms and can remain in the blood for several months afterward. It can also appear in individuals who live in close contact with many people (as in institutions) and in laboratory technicians who work with blood products. Rarely, patients with certain forms of leukemia show a positive AU test.

AUTOMATED REAGIN, see *Syphilis*

A–Z, see *Pregnancy*

B$_{12}$, see *Schilling*

BABINSKI, see *Reflex*

BALANCE, see *Cerebellum*

BALLISTOCARDIOGRAM (BCG)

Ballistocardiography screens heart function indirectly by measuring the vibration of the entire body as a consequence of the heartbeat. The patient lies motionless on a special bed or platform connected to instruments that record the slightest movement of the bed. The movement of blood through the body, caused by the heartbeat, sets off a tiny vibration in the body that can be detected when the patient is lying perfectly still. This motion is amplified electrically and recorded as waves on a chart. It is interesting to note that the secondary motion of the body caused by heart movements is about the same in a human as it is in a mouse or a whale.

When performed: While primarily a research test, ballistocardiography is also used to help diagnose heart disease before symptoms appear. It can help measure the result of treatment of heart disease, especially the effect of certain drugs on the heart.

Normal values: Although normal values change with age, certain types of waves indicate the condition of the heart. Unfortunately, there are several different standards of "normal," depending mostly on the experience of the cardiologist performing and interpreting the test.

Abnormal values: Certain categories of abnormal values are obvious to the trained cardiologist; but if three different cardiologists read the same ballistocardiogram, there could be three different interpretations. The test, however, can be helpful in rare instances when a specific diagnosis has been impossible to make.

BARBITURATES

When there is a suspicion of accidental or suicidal ingestion of barbiturates (Seconal, Nembutal, phenobarbital) in an unconscious patient, blood, serum, or plasma (usually from a vein) is examined to ascertain the barbiturate level. Urine can also be examined for barbiturates as a rapid screening test. Body organs such as the liver store barbiturates, and the level can be detected from a **Biopsy**.

When performed: When a patient is unconscious and the cause is unknown; to distinguish the comatose state from that due to other causes such as diabetic coma and alcoholic and/or tranquilizer intoxication; to aid in deciding the type of therapy for the unconscious patient; in medical-legal situations of suspected drug abuse.

Normal values: Normally there are no barbiturates in the blood.

Abnormal values: Any barbiturate in the blood greater than 0.01 mg per 100 ml is considered dangerous. It is important to know the kinds and amounts of barbiturates in the blood, because a small amount of a quick-acting barbiturate such as Nembutal or Seconal is far more deadly than a larger amount of a longer-acting barbiturate such as phenobarbital. Certain drugs such as aspirin, aminophylline, and some antibiotics can interfere with the test technique and cause erroneous results.

BARIUM ENEMA, see *Radiography*

BARIUM SWALLOW, see *Radiography*

BARR BODIES, see *Chromatin*

BASAL BODY TEMPERATURE, see *Body Temperature*

BASAL METABOLIC RATE (BMR)

The basal metabolic rate (BMR) is primarily a measure of thyroid function. The patient fasts prior to the test, and the test is performed when the patient is as relaxed as possible, both physically and mentally. The patient breathes into a machine that measures the body's oxygen consumption and the calories expended while at rest.

When performed: The test is used when there is a suspicion of endocrine disease or when metabolic processes must be studied but the patient's iodine intake or exposure precludes the more precise chemical tests (see **Thyroid Function**). Iodine compounds used in some diagnostic tests can stay in the body for five years or more.

Normal values: Normal values range from −15% to +15% of the amount of oxygen a person of a specific age, height, and weight typically uses at rest.

Abnormal values: The BMR may be elevated (the patient uses more than a normal amount of oxygen) in hyperthyroidism, acromegaly, diabetes insipidus, Cushing's disease, leukemia, pulmonary and cardiovascular disease, acidosis, and anxiety. Tremor, shivering, and generalized movement can accelerate the

BMR and give false high values. The BMR is lower than normal with hypothyroidism (cretinism).

BASE EXCESS OR DEFICIT, see *Bicarbonate*

BAYLEY SCALE, see *Motor Development*

BCG, see *Ballistocardiogram*

BECK DEPRESSION INVENTORY, see *Depression*

BELLAK, see *Thematic Apperception*

BENCE-JONES PROTEIN

Bence-Jones protein is a nonalbumin protein that is rarely found in the urine. (Albumin is the most common form of protein that is found in the urine; any measurable protein in the urine is abnormal.) Bence-Jones protein is a test primarily for multiple myeloma (a cancer of the plasma cells usually arising in bone marrow). In one out of five patients with multiple myeloma (myelomatosis), detection of Bence-Jones protein (the globulin that comes from the cancerous cells) in the urine is the only way to diagnose the disease. A urine sample is examined by adding an antiserum.

When performed: When there is a suspicion of multiple myeloma; when there are many unexplained infections; when there is unexplainable bleeding into tissues.

Normal values: There may be a very slight trace of Bence-Jones protein in the urine, but it is usually not measurable.

Abnormal values: Bence-Jones protein is primarily associated with multiple myeloma. It may also be found in cases of Waldenström's macroglobulinemia, where lymphocytes (white blood cells) as well as plasma cells are produced in excess numbers. The Bradshaw test, a newer test somewhat similar to Bence-Jones, is positive in 95% of cases of multiple myeloma.

BENDER GESTALT, see *Visual Motor Perception*

BENDER-PURDUE REFLEX, see *Reflex*

BENZIDINE, see *Occult Blood*

BERIBERI, see *Thiamin*

BICARBONATE (HCO₃)

Bicarbonate (sometimes called carbonates) is the most important buffer compound in the blood. A buffer keeps the **pH** (acid-base balance) of the blood at its proper strength. Bicarbonate is a blood electrolyte that works hand in hand with carbonic acid (from which it is derived as part of the metabolism of food) to help regulate blood pH. There is 20 times as much bicarbonate in the blood as carbonic acid; thus the normal pH is slightly alkaline.

Bicarbonate is easily regulated by the kidney, which excretes it when there is an excess and holds it back when needed; the amount of carbon dioxide in the blood, and the amount breathed out by the lungs, also controls bicarbonate levels. If bicarbonate is lost from the body because of a kidney problem, diarrhea, or other disease, a state of acidosis (too much acid in the blood) exists.

In most instances the bicarbonate concentration is determined by testing for the total amount of carbon dioxide, but at times bicarbonate itself becomes a valuable measurement. The "standard bicarbonate" or base excess or deficit may also be measured, but this is rarely done in practice. Blood is taken from a vein and the serum is tested.

When performed: As a verification of other tests such as the blood gases (carbon dioxide, oxygen, and hydrogen) and the pH; when there is some doubt as to the exact state of the blood pH; to differentiate the type of kidney disease, toxic coma, and certain lung problems.

Normal values: Blood bicarbonate levels normally range from 24 to 26 mEq per liter.

Abnormal values: Bicarbonate is usually increased when there is severe vomiting, when excessive bicarbonatelike products are ingested (antacid preparations for ulcers or burning stomach); when diuretic and steroid drugs are used, and when difficult breathing prevents the release of proper amounts of carbon dioxide. Blood bicarbonate is decreased moderately with rapid breathing (when excessive carbon dioxide is exhaled) and with liver disease; it is decreased markedly with aspirin or other toxic chemical poisoning, with kidney disease, and with diarrhea.

BILE DUCT VISUALIZATION, see *Radiography*

BILIRUBIN

Bilirubin is a gold-colored pigment waste product of the body. It is formed mostly from the hemoglobin in red blood cells when they break down at the end of their usual life span (four months). Every day about 7 to 8 g (a teaspoon and a half) of hemoglobin is released from dying red blood cells to make 250 mg of bilirubin. Bilirubin then becomes part of the bile fluid that goes from the liver to the gall bladder to the intestines; almost all of it is normally eliminated by the bowels.

Excessive production or decreased excretion of bilirubin increases the minute normal amounts in the blood, and its unique color, when increased, causes yellow jaundice in the skin and the whites of the eyes. Before it is acted upon by the liver, bilirubin is attached to albumin protein molecules in the blood; in this state it is called indirect bilirubin. After it is acted upon by the liver, the portion no longer bound to proteins is called direct bilirubin. The sum of the two equals the total bilirubin.

Blood is taken from a vein and the serum or plasma is examined. Bilirubin is also measured in the urine (only direct bilirubin is excreted, causing a dark color). Shaking urine in a glass tube will change the normal white color of the foam to a dark yellow or brown if bilirubin is present. Amniotic fluid (the water around the fetus during pregnancy) may also be tested for excess bilirubin (it is normally present in tiny amounts and decreases throughout pregnancy).

When performed: The test is performed primarily to distinguish different forms of liver disease, especially liver cell disease from bile duct obstruction such as from gallstones. It can also help determine the cause of certain anemias. When a patient has gray-white or colorless bowel movements, the bilirubin is measured to ascertain the cause.

Normal values: The total serum bilirubin runs from 0.2 to 1.5 mg per 100 ml. The direct bilirubin usually measures from 0.1 to 0.4 mg per 100 ml; the indirect bilirubin runs about the same but may be slightly higher and still be normal. The urine normally contains no bilirubin. Amniotic fluid usually contains a trace of bilirubin.

Abnormal values: Total bilirubin (both direct and indirect) is increased with liver cirrhosis. When something blocks the flow of bile, such as a gall stone or cancer of the pancreas, the total and direct bilirubin is increased, but the indirect bilirubin usually stays within its normal range. Liver disease from Thorazine and other tranquilizers as well as drugs such as male hormones, some antibiotics, and certain arthritic pain products can cause elevated direct bilirubin; usually the indirect bilirubin stays normal. In contrast, in certain anemias where blood cells break easily such as erythroblastosis fetalis (the anemia most often caused by Rh problems), the total serum bilirubin and the indirect bilirubin are elevated, but the direct bilirubin stays normal. As red blood cells are destroyed, the bilirubin increases in amniotic fluid, and this is a way of following the course of the disease. Fasting or low caloric diet causes a marked rise in serum bilirubin in 24 hours.

BIOFEEDBACK, see *Electroencephalogram*

BIOMICROSCOPE, see *Fluorescein Eye Stain*

BIOPSY

Biopsy is the removal of a piece of tissue from the body for detailed, usually microscopic, examination. Examination of isolated cells such as blood cells or those obtained for a bone marrow test or Pap smear (see **Cytology**) are forms of a biopsy. Most often, however, a small piece of tissue is excised with a scalpel. (If the lesion is small, as are most skin growths, the entire mass is removed.) The specimen is sliced to extreme thinness (microtomy), stained, and examined through the microscope.

In needle biopsy, a fine needle is inserted into a body organ, tissue, or suspected lesion and a minute piece is sucked into the needle tip for microscopic examination. This is usually performed under the fluoroscope so as to be precise about the location of the specimen. In most instances a local anesthetic is used. Needle biopsies of the breast, liver, spleen, pancreas, kidney, and lung are regularly performed. Biopsy of the prostate may be obtained during cystoscopy (use of an instrument that allows a direct view of the urethra and bladder). In general, the result of a biopsy of a tumor is reported as benign (noncancerous) or malignant (cancerous). A biopsy may also reveal an infection or foreign body as the cause of the lesion.

When performed: Whenever a suspicious lesion is seen (either directly on the skin or in a body cavity), felt (as in the breast), or noted (by X-ray); whenever there is suspected disease in an organ (such as the liver or lung) that cannot be diagnosed.

Normal values: The very existence of a lesion usually contradicts a normal value, but there are various skin growths such as birthmarks that are not disease related.

Abnormal values: Any biopsy showing pathological cells is considered abnormal. Benign cells can be pathological, or disease related, even if they are not cancerous.

BLACKY PICTURES, see *Thematic Apperception*

BLADDER STONE, see *Urinary Tract Calculus*

BLEEDING AND CLOTTING TIME

Although essentially two different tests, bleeding and clotting time are invariably performed together as if they were one. They are crude measures of hemostasis (how quickly bleeding is stopped by normal body responses). More specifically, bleeding time is primarily an indication of the condition of the blood vessels (principally the capillaries) and an indication of platelet function. In addition to clotting factors, the test measures how well and how quickly small arteries and veins will constrict and close off to stop bleeding when injured. Clotting time is a generalized indication of the effectiveness of the many factors within the fluid blood itself (as opposed to the blood vessels) to bring about coagulation (clotting).

The original technique of nicking the earlobe or a fingertip is still used occasionally to measure bleeding time. However, the preferred technique (Ivy bleeding time) is to apply a standard amount of pressure around the upper arm with a blood pressure cuff and then to make two incisions 10 mm (about 7/16″) long and 1 mm (1/32″) deep on the lower arm. Blotting paper is touched to the cut every 30 seconds until the bleeding stops, at which point the time is noted.

In tests of clotting time, blood is usually drawn from a vein and placed in several narrow glass tubes. Sometimes the tubes are broken apart; sometimes they are tilted. In either case, the time is noted when the blood visibly clots (the cells go from a liquid to a solid state).

When performed: The test is used when there are unusual bleeding tendencies (either inherited or caused by drugs or other diseases); when liver disease is suspected, and whenever a patient is to have a surgical procedure or extensive dental work. The clotting time alone may be measured as a guide to dosage when a patient receives heparin as part of anticoagulant therapy; it may also be used as a test of platelet function (see **Platelet Count**).

Normal values: Bleeding time usually averages 5 minutes; however, bleeding times of up to 10 minutes are still considered within normal limits by some laboratories. Clotting time usually ranges from 6 to 16 minutes.

Abnormal values: Longer than usual bleeding time generally indicates thrombocytopenia (a decrease in the normal amount of blood platelets, which are essential for clotting). It can also mean that the platelets, although normal in number, are not functioning properly. Bleeding and clotting time together are prolonged when there are coagulation defects—either absence of the multiple clot-causing factors normally in blood or interference with one or more of these factors (such as when a patient is given heparin). The clotting time alone is not a specific diagnostic test. It is usually (though not always) increased with hemophilia. Taking large doses of aspirin can cause increased bleeding and clotting times, as can uremia (a form of kidney failure where the by-products of proteins cannot filter through the kidney) and certain kinds of leukemia.

BLIND SPOT, see *Visual Field*

BLOOD ACIDITY, see *pH*

BLOOD CELL DIFFERENTIAL

Changes in the amounts of *each type* of **White blood cell** (leukocyte) and changes in the size and shape of **Red blood cells** (erythrocytes) can be of greater importance than changes in the total white and red blood cell counts. Particularly, ascertaining changes in the proportions of the different kinds of white blood cells helps to define different disease processes. The blood cell differential test also distinguishes abnormalities in red blood cells (such as sickling, different forms of anemia, insufficient iron) and will show malaria if present. A drop of blood is taken from the fingertip, earlobe, or heel; or a drop of venous blood taken for other tests may be used. The blood is stained and then examined through a microscope by a hematologist or trained technician. No machine can perform this test.

When performed: When there is an infectious process, an allergy, or a parasitic infestation; with suspicion of any blood disease such as anemia or leukemia.

Normal values: Usually each of the different kinds of white blood cells are found in the following proportions:

Neutrophils: 65% total, with 58% mature neutrophils and 7% young neutrophils (neutrophils are the primary cells that ingest and destroy microorganisms and other toxic disease-producing substances).

Lymphocytes: 27% (lymphocytes represent antibody activity in producing immunity to disease).

Monocytes: 5% (while thought of as old lymphocytes, they represent chronic disease processes in the body).

Eosinophils: 2% (eosinophils are related to allergies and parasitic infestations).

Basophils: 1% (the role of the basophil is still not clearly understood).

Abnormal values: An increased proportion of neutrophils usually indicates poisoning, cancer, hemorrhage, or an infectious process (there are a few exceptions; for reasons still unknown, a virus infection, typhoid fever, and malaria do not cause the expected increase in neutrophils). When most of the neutrophils are young, elevated levels usually reflect leukemia. A decreased amount of neutrophils is seen with spleen disorders, lupus erythematosus, vitamin B_{12} and/or folic acid deficiency, and bone marrow damage from drugs or X-rays. Typhoid and malaria are two infections that cause a decrease in neutrophils.

Lymphocytes are increased primarily after radiation exposure and in hepatitis, herpes simplex and herpes zoster (shingles), infectious mononucleosis, syphilis, and leukemia. They are decreased in lupus erythematosus and other conditions where there is reduced immunity to disease.

Monocytes are increased with tuberculosis, cancers, anemias, rickettsial diseases (such as Rocky Mountain spotted fever), and typhoid. A decrease in monocytes is rarely seen.

Eosinophils are increased with asthma, hay fever, and similar conditions, and especially with worm and other parasite invasion. They are decreased with alcohol intoxication.

Basophils may be increased with leukemias and adrenal disease and are sometimes missing with hyperthyroidism and allergies.

BLOOD COUNT, see *Red Blood Cell*; *White Blood Cell*

BLOOD CULTURE, see *Culture*

BLOOD DONOR HEPATITIS, see *Isocitric Dehydrogenase*

BLOOD ELECTROLYTES, see *Bicarbonate*; *Chloride*; *Potassium*; *Sodium*

BLOOD FATS, see *Lipids*

BLOOD GASES, see *Carbon Dioxide*; *Oxygen*

BLOOD MATCHING, see *Typing and Cross-Matching*

BLOOD POOL SCAN, see *Nuclear Scanning*

BLOOD PRESSURE

The term "blood pressure" generally refers to the pressure in the arteries as opposed to the veins. To take one's blood pressure is to measure the pressure (tension) of the blood within the artery walls. (Pressures in the capillaries and veins are quite different.) The end result is derived from a number of factors: the force of each heartbeat, the elasticity or resilience of the walls of the artery, the amount of blood flowing through the arteries at any one time, the viscosity (thickness) of the blood, the number of molecules of various substances (such as protein and sodium) in the blood, the amount of certain hormones and enzymes (such as adrenalin from the adrenal gland and renin from the kidney) circulating in the blood, and the functioning of the autonomic or sympathetic nervous system (over which a person has no direct control) in response to changes in posture, stressful situations, and other stimuli.

The blood pressure is altered during every heartbeat, reaching its highest point when the heart muscle is most contracted (forcing blood into the arteries) and its lowest point when the heart muscle relaxes after each heartbeat. The heart muscle contraction is medically called systole, and the highest point of one's blood pressure is known as systolic. The momentary resting phase of the heart is called diastole, and the low point of one's blood pressure is known as diastolic. The difference between these two pressures is called the pulse pressure.

The measurement of blood pressure is recorded by noting how high in millimeters (mm) applied pressure will cause a column of mercury (Hg) to rise on a measuring instrument. A cuff or sleeve is wrapped around an extremity (most commonly the upper arm); air is pumped into the cuff to apply a counterpressure to all the tissues surrounding the artery (skin, muscles, etc.). By reading the level of counterpressure on an air pressure dial gauge or directly observing how high the mercury rises, the physician can note when the artery collapses (similar to applying a tourniquet and then releasing the pressure to allow the artery to fill normally); at that point the pressure being applied just exceeds the pressure within the artery. Collapse of the artery is most commonly noted by listening for the cessation of the pulse through a stethoscope placed on the inside of the arm in front of the elbow or by feeling for the pulse until the examiner can no longer feel the beat.

When sufficient pressure is applied around the arm to collapse the artery, the pulse will no longer be heard or felt, giving the systolic blood pressure reading. As outside pressure from the cuff is lessened, the pulse can be heard or felt the instant the artery pressure exceeds that of the surrounding cuff (again the measure of the systolic pressure). The pulse will be heard or felt as long as sufficient pressure is applied from the outside to cause the blood pulsations to rebound off the artery walls. When the outside pressure is low enough so there is no measurable resistance against the artery wall, the pulse will no longer be heard (it will still be felt); this point is noted for the diastolic pressure measurement. Today there are electronic instruments that translate the pulse sounds into light impulses or noises, which are much easier to record.

It is important to measure blood pressure in both arms and both legs; to measure it while the patient is standing, sitting, and lying down; and most of all to measure it when the patient is as relaxed as possible. Most physicians measure blood pressure at the onset of an examination, again about halfway through and as the last procedure (when the patient is most likely to be at ease). Recently, doctors have asked patients to measure their own blood pressure at home (or have a family member test it) during various times of the day and to note activities at the time in order to arrive at the most usual reading. Blood pressure readings must be abnormal on three different days before a diagnosis of hypertension can be made.

Venous blood pressure as opposed to arterial blood pressure is recorded directly by using a manometer, a thin glass tube with measurement markings connected to a needle. The needle is placed inside a vein in the arm, which is kept at heart level (it may also be placed in a neck vein, with the patient lying down); the actual rise of blood in the tube is noted. Vein pressure can be estimated by observing the veins on the back of the hand when the arm is raised. Normally the veins collapse when the hand reaches heart level; neck veins usually collapse when the patient is in a sitting position.

When performed: Arterial blood pressure is routinely measured during a physical examination to detect early stages of hypertension (high blood pressure), a condition that exists in one out of every ten Americans. It is also followed closely in patients who are overweight; patients who have thyroid and other hormone diseases, kidney diseases, or lung diseases; and during pregnancy (see **Rollover**). During surgical procedures the blood pressure is monitored constantly as a guide to the patient's condition, especially to check for blood loss.

Venous blood pressure is measured primarily in heart disease to determine which side of the heart is in difficulty. It is also measured when blood transfusions are given to make sure the patient does not receive too much blood (which can cause congestion of the lungs) as well as when intravenous fluids are administered to patients in diabetic coma.

Normal values: The most generalized figures given for arterial blood pressure are 120/80, which means the systolic pressure is 120 mm Hg and the diastolic pressure is 80 mm Hg when a person is at rest and relaxed. But blood pressure seems to rise naturally as people get older. Even with age, however, the diastolic pressure should not rise as much as the systolic. A consistent blood pressure of greater than 140/85, regardless of age, should be thought of as a warning sign. Venous blood pressure normally ranges from 40 to 80 mm Hg. The pulse pressure averages 40 mm Hg.

Abnormal values: In general, a systolic blood pressure reading over 150 mm Hg and/or a diastolic blood pressure reading over 90 mm Hg is considered evidence of hypertension. Three out of four people with high blood pressure readings (excluding those obtained erroneously) have essential hypertension (caused by some direct body dysfunction); one out of four cases of hypertension have a secondary cause that can be diagnosed, such as kidney disease, connective tissue disease, nervous system involvement, lung disease, or hormonal problems. Certain drugs such as those used for asthma can cause high blood pressure readings.

High blood pressure is more a cause of heart disease than a result of heart problems. When blood pressure is elevated in the arms but normal or low in the legs, or when blood pressure in the right arm is greater than in the left, it usually indicates coarctation (constriction) of the aorta. Hypotension, or low blood pressure, most commonly occurs when a person moves from a sitting to a standing position (postural or orthostatic hypotension). It may also be caused by diuretic and other antihypertensive drugs, by many tranquilizers, by certain Parkinson-type diseases, and, of course, by shock or severe bleeding.

A major cause of erroneous arterial blood pressure readings is faulty measurement technique. Putting the cuff on wrong, not inflating the cuff properly, and failing to hear the proper pulse sounds (either because of inattentiveness or because of other distracting noises) are the three most common reasons for erroneous, usually elevated, blood pressure readings. Performing a single test, on one arm, at the onset of an examination can also lead to inaccurate high blood pressure readings. Failure to take into account any apprehensiveness on the part of a patient will invariably give false results.

Venous blood pressure rises primarily with heart conditions such as right-sided heart failure or heart valve damage to the point that blood cannot easily enter the heart chambers. A rapid fall in venous pressure usually indicates internal bleeding such as from an ulcer.

BLOOD TYPE, see *Agglutination*

BLOOD UREA NITROGEN, see *Urea Nitrogen*

BMR, see *Basal Metabolic Rate*

BODY SCANNING, see *Computerized Tomography*

BODY TEMPERATURE

Although a rise in the temperature of the body is usually an indication of disease, especially infection, body temperature also rises slightly during the menstrual cycle. The basal body temperature test indicates the time of ovulation (when the ovum or egg is released from the ovary ready for fertilization or pregnancy). The body temperature is taken each morning on arising (usually by mouth) and recorded. It usually remains slightly below normal (normal is 98.6° F, or 37° C) until ovulation occurs, when it rises to normal or slightly above and stays elevated until menstruation. Thus, if a woman is having difficulty becoming pregnant, the couple is told to wait for the temperature to rise before having intercourse. The test can, of course, also be used as a contraceptive guide to show when conception would be impossible. The basal temperature test is used in conjunction with the Pap test (see **Cytology**) to study the menstrual cycle phase.

Temperature may also be measured in the urine. There are times when a patient has a persistent high fever, yet no body pathology is detected. Measuring the temperature of the urine immediately after it is passed will indicate which patients have a false high temperature—that is, which patients are employing devices to deliberately raise the temperature of the thermometer.

When performed: The basal body temperature is measured when patients have fertility problems; when chemical contraception is obviated; and when gynecological problems are suspected. The urinary temperature test is used when patients are suspected of faking fever.

Normal values: Normal body temperature is usually between 98° and 99° F, or around 37° C; there is normally a 1° rise in temperature at the time of ovulation.

Abnormal values: Any elevation of body temperature greater than 100° F, failure of the body temperature to rise about 1° in the midmenstrual cycle, and a difference of more than 1° between body and urine temperature are all considered abnormal.

BOECK'S SARCOID, see *Kveim*

BONE MARROW

Red and white blood cells and platelets are produced in the bone marrow. When a disease process affects the bone marrow, there is either an increase or a reduction of these essential blood elements. Also, depending on the nature of the disease, **Iron** may be increased in, or lost from, the bone marrow. A tiny amount of bone marrow can be aspirated (withdrawn) for examination with a syringe and special needle. The most common sites for bone marrow aspiration are the crest of the hip bone and the sternum (breast bone). Bone marrow may also be cultured for infection (see **Culture**).

When performed: When leukemia, certain anemias, blood diseases such as hemolysis (self-destruction of red blood cells) or polycythemia (too many red blood cells), drug toxicity, or tumor growths such as lymphoma, myelofibrosis, and multiple myeloma are suspected; to follow the effectiveness of therapy in these diseases.

Normal values: A normal bone marrow specimen contains 15 different kinds of cells in varying stages of growth and in varying amounts. Normally, a small amount of iron is found in the marrow (detected using a special stain). Examination and determination of the normalcy of the different kinds of cells and the amount of iron must be made by a hematologist.

Abnormal values: Evidence of red cell destruction, presence of sickle or other diseased cells, absence of normal cells, and excess of diseased cells are all considered abnormal. Iron absence is found with iron deficiency anemia (usually due to blood loss); an increase in iron is seen with pernicious and hemolytic anemia and anemia caused by infection.

BONE SCAN, see *Nuclear Scanning*

BOWEL BLEEDING, see *Occult Blood*

BRADSHAW, see *Bence-Jones Protein*

BRAIN SCAN, see *Nuclear Scanning*

BRAIN WAVE, see *Electroencephalogram*

BREAST CANCER, see *T-Antigen*

BREATH ALCOHOL, see *Alcohol*

BREATHING, see *Smell Function*

BRODIE-TRENDELENBERG, see *Tourniquet Test for Varicose Veins*

BROMIDES

In the days before tranquilizers, bromides were sometimes prescribed for sedation, but they rarely are anymore. However, some medicines available without prescriptions still contain bromides (Sleep-Eze, Sominex), and patients sometimes dose themselves to excess. Bromide drugs can cause mental manifestations imitating schizophrenia. Blood is collected from a vein and the serum is examined. The urine can also be examined for bromides.

When performed: The test is one of many usually performed on an unconscious patient when there is no known cause for coma. It is also performed when excess intake of bromides is suspected and on patients who are confused or appear to be psychotic, especially when such behavior is new.

Normal values: Normally there is no measurable amount of bromide in the blood serum and none in the urine.

Abnormal values: When a toxic amount of bromide has been ingested, more than 150 mg of bromide per 100 ml of serum is usually detected.

BROMSULPHALEIN (BSP)

The bromsulphalein (BSP) retention test is used primarily to evaluate liver function when jaundice is *not* present. BSP is a dye that is injected into a vein after the patient has fasted for at least 12 hours (water is permitted). A normal working liver will immediately take up almost all the injected dye from the blood and secrete it into the bile. After 45 minutes a blood sample is taken (from a different vein), and the amount of dye still remaining in the serum is measured. The dye is irritating and must be injected very carefully so that it does not seep around the vein under the skin, where it can cause tissue damage. It can also cause severe allergic shock in susceptible people. BSP is being replaced by a new dye, indocyanine green (ICG), which does not seem to cause irritation or allergy.

When performed: The test is used when there is a suspicion of liver disease or some related condition of the gall bladder or bile ducts. It is primarily a screening test, since it does not reveal any specific diagnosis, and is used mostly when other, more precise liver function tests cannot be employed. The test is sometimes performed to follow the progress of a known liver condition during treatment.

Normal values: After the 45-minute period following injection of the dye, the blood normally retains less than 5% of that dye. With advancing age, up to 10% of the dye normally may still be found in the blood. A normal value, however, does not positively exclude liver disease.

Abnormal values: When there is liver disease, the blood may still have 80% of BSP after 45 minutes. Excess BSP retention in the blood can also be caused by gall bladder inflammation, intestinal hemorrhage, obesity, and drugs such as barbiturates, oral contraceptives and other estrogens, medication to help lower cholesterol levels, and phenolphthalein (in Ex-Lax and some other laxatives). If albumin (a normal serum protein) is lower than normal, an artificially low BSP will result.

BRONCHOGRAPHY, see *Radiography*

BRONCHOSCOPY, see *Endoscopy*

BRUCELLOSIS, see *Agglutination*

BSP, see *Bromsulphalein*

BUCCAL SMEAR, see *Chromatin*

BUFFER, see *Bicarbonate*

BUN, see *Urea Nitrogen*

C, see *Complement*

C-1 ESTERASE INHIBITOR, see *Complement*

CALCIFEROL, see *Vitamin D*

CALCITONIN

Calcitonin is a hormone produced by the thyroid gland. Its principal task seems to be to help the body get rid of excess **Calcium.** It acts in opposition to the parathyroid gland hormone in that it slows down the release of calcium from the bones to the serum. Blood is taken from a vein and the serum is tested. Calcitonin from salmon is even more potent in humans than human calcitonin and is used to treat certain bone disease.

When performed: When X-rays show the bones to be losing minerals; when thyroid cancer or certain adrenal tumors are suspected; to verify high levels of calcium in the blood.

Normal values: From 5 to 300 pg per ml (usually less than 400 pg per ml) is considered normal.

Abnormal values: Calcitonin levels are increased with certain thyroid cancers, stomach cancers, anemia, and kidney disease.

CALCIUM

There are approximately two pounds of calcium in the body at all times, almost all in the bones and teeth. About 0.03 ounce of calcium is taken in each day in a normal diet. This is the bare minimum required to fulfill the body's regular needs, because 80% of ingested calcium is excreted (in urine and sweat and through the bowels). Calcium is needed to maintain many body processes such as muscle contraction and nerve transmission, to keep cells from being destroyed, and to ensure that blood will clot.

The body's calcium need and use are controlled by the hormone from the parathyroid glands (four separate, tiny glands buried within the thyroid gland but distinctly different from it) and almost as much by the amount of phosphorus and vitamin D in the body (see **Alkaline Phosphatase**; **Phosphorus**). When there is an excess of parathyroid hormone, calcium increases in the blood and phosphorus decreases; with insufficient parathyroid hormone, the opposite occurs. The thyroid gland exerts a serum-lowering effect on calcium through the production of a unique hormone called **Calcitonin.**

Three different forms of calcium are in the blood: the ionized or active form, which comprises approximately half the total amount; 45% in a form attached to the serum protein albumin; and a form attached to phosphates, which comprises about 5% of the total. The usual test for calcium measures all three forms and is called the total calcium (there are special tests to measure only the ionized portion). Blood calcium is measured in the serum from venous blood. It is also measured in the urine (Sulkowitch test), in the feces, and in the spinal fluid.

When performed: The test is used primarily when there are suspected abnormalities of the parathyroid gland; when there are mysterious symptoms such as memory problems, unusual sleepiness, or nerve and muscle problems; and, in contrast, when there is excessive muscle irritability. When a patient has difficulty swallowing, tongue problems, or certain forms of deafness, calcium levels in the blood may aid in discovering the cause. Other gland dysfunctions such as a lack of adrenal hormones or too much thyroid hormone may be diagnosed by testing for calcium. The test is also used when there is suspicion of vitamin D poisoning or unexplained bleeding and to differentiate various bone diseases, including the unique bone problems of women after the menopause.

Normal values: Normal values in serum range from 8.5 to 10.5 mg per 100 ml (4.25 to 5.25 mEq per liter); in urine, no more than 150 mg in a 24-hour sample; in feces, about 800 mg a day (depending on diet); and in spinal fluid, 4 to 5 mg per 100 ml.

Abnormal values: Serum calcium is increased in hyperparathyroidism, certain bone tumors, and rarefaction or demineralization of bone (osteoporosis); adrenal disease; hyperthyroidism; when too much vitamin D or milk is taken; when too much antacid medication (usually for ulcers) is consumed; when diuretics are taken; and in rare lung diseases. Serum calcium is decreased when the parathyroid gland is inactive or if that gland has been accidentally removed during thyroid surgery; when there is insufficient vitamin D or when vitamin D cannot be absorbed; with kidney disease and certain bone diseases such as rickets; and in nutritional problems when insufficient calcium is eaten or absorbed. When serum calcium levels are lower than normal, total serum proteins (especially albumin) must be evaluated; decreased albumin will give a decreased calcium value (see **Albumin/Globulin**).

Calcium levels in the urine fairly well reflect serum calcium levels, but they are increased when patients are taking certain diuretic drugs (which cause decreased levels in serum). Calcium is increased in feces when there are problems with intestinal absorption. Calcium levels are increased in the spinal fluid with tuberculous meningitis.

New tests are now available for measuring parathyroid hormone directly.

CALORIC

The caloric test is so named because it uses differences in temperature as the basis for diagnosing ear nerve damage that can cause dizziness.

Dizziness or vertigo can also accompany hearing loss, vision problems, brain disease, or alcoholism. Patients describe feelings of turning, twirling (or things around them twirling), and faintness. Vertigo is most often a result of disease to the vestibular part of the nerve that allows hearing; the vestibular part controls balance. In the caloric test, one teaspoon of ice water is instilled in the ear canal with a rubber syringe (similar to the technique used when washing wax out of the ear). This should cause nystagmus (the eyes move quickly away from the ice water and then slowly back). If nystagmus does not occur, two more teaspoons of ice water are used. Should the eyes still fail to move, four and then eight teaspoons of ice water are used.

At times hot water is used as well as ice water. The hot water should cause an opposite eye movement pattern from the ice water. Performing the test with both hot and cold temperatures will give more accurate results. As a confirmation for vertigo, the Romberg test is used. The patient stands with feet together and eyes closed; with vertigo the patient will tend to fall to one side.

When performed: Primarily when there is dizziness or fainting, especially after ear injury or in ear disease; whenever impaired hearing exists; with patients taking certain antibiotic drugs and with anemias; when psychological problems are suspected.

Normal values: Nystagmus should occur after one teaspoon of water is instilled in the ear canal.

Abnormal values: If nystagmus does not appear until after two or more teaspoons of ice water are placed in the ear, the ear nerve may be diseased but the possibility of cure exists. If eight teaspoons of ice water in the ear do not produce nystagmus, it may be assumed that the nerve is permanently damaged.

Vertigo can be caused by any disease or injury that affects the vestibular nerve as well as damage inflicted by many antibiotic drugs (usually when given in large doses for long periods of time). Atherosclerosis of the blood supply to the ear, cholesteotomas (growths), and certain poisons can also cause vertigo.

CANCER RESPONSIVENESS TO HORMONES, see *Estrogen Receptor*

CAPILLARY FRAGILITY (Rumpel-Leede)

In a number of diseases of blood vessels—such as thrombocytopenia (decreased thrombocytes or platelets needed for clotting), disorders of platelet function, scurvy, and purpura—the small blood vessels near the skin surface become very fragile. In the capillary fragility test, a blood pressure cuff is placed on the forearm and inflated until it is approximately midway between the diastolic and systolic pressure—usually from 80 to 100 mm of mercury (see **Blood Pressure**). This pressure is maintained for five to ten minutes. The cuff is removed and the arm is inspected for the amount of petechiae (small hemorrhages) that have appeared under the skin in a premarked area.

When performed: As one of many tests to determine hemostatic function (blood clotting and blood vessel structure).

Normal values: Normally the cuff pressure will not produce petechiae. For some unknown reason, women with red hair are sometimes more sensitive and have a slightly positive reaction without any disease condition.

Abnormal values: The appearance of multiple petechiae indicates weakness of the tiny blood vessels and/or a platelet defect.

CARBONATES, see *Bicarbonate*

CARBON DIOXIDE (CO_2)

Carbon dioxide (CO_2) and water are end products of oxygen metabolic processes. Carbon dioxide's primary route of elimination is through the lungs (during respiration the blood gives off CO_2 and picks up oxygen); a small amount of CO_2 is changed into bicarbonates and is excreted in the urine. The depth and rapidity of a person's breathing help to control the blood CO_2 levels.

There are several different ways to measure carbon dioxide in the blood. The oldest and probably the most common test (although it is considered the least precise) measures the *carbon dioxide combining power*. A more accurate evaluation is obtained by measuring the *carbon dioxide content*; when performed with the **pH** test, it will also demonstrate the exact amounts of free bicarbonate and carbonic acid in the blood. The preferred method of evaluation is testing for *carbon dioxide tension*, or PCO_2 (sometimes called partial pressure or carbonic acid concentration).

Regardless of how CO_2 is determined, the primary purpose of the test is to measure ventilation, or how well air moves in and out of the lungs. A secondary purpose is to determine what is affecting the acid-base balance or pH (acidity or alkalinity) of the blood, which is an extremely important and very sensitive reflection of potentially disastrous bodily disorders. Blood is taken from either an artery or a vein in a special syringe to avoid any contact with air, and the serum is tested.

When performed: Whenever there are respiratory problems; whenever there is suspicion of acidosis (the pH of the blood too low) or alkalosis (the pH too high), both of which are usually brought about by metabolic or respiratory disorders; when a patient has suffered severe injuries, is in coma, or is severely disoriented; when there are severe muscle cramps, severe vomiting, or diarrhea.

Normal values: Carbon dioxide tension (PCO_2) normally ranges from 35 to 45 mm Hg in arterial blood (slightly lower in women) and 38 to 50 mm Hg in venous blood; CO_2 content, from 19 to 25 mM per liter in arterial blood and 22 to 30 mM per liter in venous blood; and CO_2 combining power, from 24 to 32 mEq per liter in arterial blood and 38 to 50 mEq per liter in venous blood.

Abnormal values: Increased carbon dioxide is found primarily in respiratory acidosis from lung conditions that prevent CO_2 from being exhaled (such as asthma, emphysema, and severe chest injuries) and during anesthesia when the patient rebreathes his own air. It is usually elevated with metabolic alkalosis caused by taking diuretic drugs, steroid hormones, or antacid preparations; with vomiting, intestinal obstruction, starvation; and with hyperactive adrenal glands. Decreased carbon dioxide is found with metabolic acidosis caused by drug poisoning (especially from aspirin and from ammonium chloride that is sold for use as a diuretic without a prescription) and with diarrhea, liver disease, kidney disease, and diabetes that is out of control. It is also lower than normal when respiratory alkalosis exists (most commonly caused by hyperventilation, or deliberate rapid breathing).

CARBOXYHEMOGLOBIN, see *Hemoglobin*

CARCINOEMBRYONIC ANTIGEN (CEA)

Originally the carcinoembryonic antigen (CEA) test was used to detect cancer of the colon, but the antigen has since been found to appear with other cancers as well (pancreas, lung, breast, and prostate). Blood is drawn from a vein and the serum is examined. Other body fluids (joint fluid, peritoneal fluid, amniotic fluid) may also be tested.

When performed: The test is performed primarily to follow the course and treatment of patients with known cancers. It is also used to determine the extent of cancer, since CEA can return to normal values following successful surgery. When a cancer patient has a checkup, the levels of carcinoembryonic antigen may rise months before new symptoms appear, alerting the doctor to the need for immediate further therapy. The test may also be performed to diagnose certain causes of jaundice.

Normal values: Levels below 2 ng per ml are not considered indicative of pathology. Carcinoembryonic antigen is found in very small amounts in many pregnant women, in infants, and in other normal individuals.

Abnormal values: A CEA greater than 5 to 10 ng per ml is found in a majority of patients with known cancer. Increased values are also found in patients with alcoholic cirrhosis, colitis, ulcers, and emphysema, and in heavy smokers. A subspecies of CEA called CEA-S is specific for gastrointestinal cancers without being elevated for other conditions.

CARDIAC CINERADIOGRAPHY, see *Radiography*

CARDIAC GLYCOSIDE, see *Digitalis Toxicity*

CARDIAC SCAN, see *Nuclear Scanning*

CARDIOGRAM, see *Electrocardiogram*

CAROTENE, see *Retinal*

CAROTID ARTERY PULSE, see *Pulse Analysis*

CAT (X-RAY), see *Computerized Tomography*

CATECHOLAMINES

Catecholamines are produced by the medulla, or central part of the adrenal gland, as opposed to the outer area or cortex, where cortisone-type hormones originate (see **Cortisol**). Epinephrine (adrenalin) and norepinephrine (noradrenalin) are the two principal catecholamine hormones. They are called pressor amines because of their ability to constrict blood vessel walls, thus elevating the blood pressure. Norepinephrine is also necessary to transmit nerve impulses in the brain.

The two catecholamines can be tested in the blood, but they are most commonly measured in the urine, along with their metabolic end products, vanillymandelic acid (VMA), homovanillic acid (HVA), and metanephrines. Recently it has been found that decreased amounts of norepinephrine in the brain cause patients to experience symptoms of depression; excessive amounts seem to be associated with manic symptoms.

When performed: When pheochromocytoma (a tumor of the adrenal gland that causes high blood pressure) is suspected; to assess adrenal function; in certain cases of depression when a specific cause cannot be found.

Normal values: Urine levels should not exceed 100 mcg per 100 ml in a 24-hour sample. A single urine sample should not exceed 15 mcg per 100 ml. Plasma epinephrine averages 20 ng per 100 ml; norepinephrine, 60 ng per 100 ml. Urine VMA should not exceed 8 mg per 100 ml in a 24-hour sample.

Abnormal values: When total urine catecholamines exceed 200 mcg per 100 ml and/or VMA is greater than 25 mg per 100 ml, disease is present, most likely pheochromocytoma. However, several other nerve tumors can cause increased values (in which case HVA is also increased), as can myasthenia gravis and muscular dystrophy. Certain drugs such as those used to treat depression, aspirin, some antibiotics, and coffee, tea, chocolates, fruits, and vanilla extract can cause false high values. Stress or exercise can increase catecholamines. Increased norepinephrine has been found in autism.

CAT SCAN, see *Computerized Tomography*

CEA, see *Carcinoembryonic Antigen*

CENTRAL VISUAL FIELD, see *Visual Field*

CEPHALIN FLOCCULATION (Cephalin-Cholesterol Flocculation)

Cephalin flocculation is used to measure liver cell function. Cephalin is a plasma lipid. It will not normally flocculate, or clump, if there are balanced levels of serum albumin and gamma globulins. When the **Albumin/Globulin** ratio is upset, the woolly-looking precipitation (flocculation) of cephalin is increased. Blood from a vein is tested. A **Thymol Turbidity** test is usually performed as a parallel check on cephalin flocculation.

When performed: As a general screening test when liver disease is suspected; to follow the progress of patients with known liver disease.

Normal values: From negative to no more than a 1-plus (very slight) flocculation is considered normal.

Abnormal values: Readings of 2-plus to 4-plus (visibly increased clumping) suggest liver disease from within the liver itself, as opposed to a bile tract obstruction.

CEREBELLUM

The cerebellum is the part of the brain that helps control balance and coordination. Loss of coordinated movements can result from cerebellum disease as well as from certain nerve conditions that cause inability to feel pressure and other sensations. The cerebellum tests help to determine if the problem is in the brain itself, as opposed to the spinal cord and its nerve extensions.

The easiest coordination test is to have the patient stand up with feet together and close his eyes; with cerebellum disease the patient tends to fall. Attempting to walk heel to toe with eyes closed is an extension of the same test. In another simple coordination test the patient may be asked to touch the tip of his nose with his finger (with the arm first extended out); the test is repeated with the eyes closed. Trying to touch the fingers in rapid succession with the thumb is another cerebellum test, as is trying to point to objects with the big toe while lying down.

When performed: In cases of ataxia (loss of muscle coordination or irregular muscle actions); when brain disease is suspected; following head injuries; to differentiate alcoholism, drug, or hysterical reactions from physical disease.

Normal values: Normally patients perform the simple tasks of coordination without difficulty.

Abnormal values: Patients with impaired coordination are unable to perform the simple movements described. Usually, only one side of the body is affected with cerebellum disease; both sides of the body are usually involved with conditions that arise from below the brain level.

CEREBRAL ANGIOGRAPHY, see *Radiography*

CEREBROSPINAL FLUID

Testing the spinal fluid—more accurately described as the cerebrospinal fluid, since it surrounds the brain as well as the spinal cord—is a valuable diagnostic aid in many nervous system diseases (infections and brain and spinal cord damage associated with injury or cancer). Many tests may be performed on the spinal fluid; the usual examination consists of measuring the pressure of the fluid within the spinal canal, observing the transparency and color of the fluid, and counting the white blood cells. The most common chemical tests performed on spinal fluid to establish or prove a diagnosis are chloride, sugar, proteins, and quantitative VDRL (Venereal Disease Research Laboratories) reactions to follow the treatment for syphilis. A small needle is placed in the back, between the lumbar (lower back) vertebrae, and the fluid is withdrawn (hence the term "lumbar puncture"). The test should not be performed when there is suspicion of increased intracranial pressure.

When performed: Following head or back injury or when such injury is suspected but not proved; when symptoms suggest brain tumor or stroke; when there is a severe infection (virus, meningitis, poliomyelitis, encephalitis) that seems to be affecting the brain or muscles; when there are suspected birth injuries.

Normal values: The spinal fluid has a normal pressure equal to 70 to 200 mm of water (in the sitting position; it is slightly lower when lying down). The fluid should be transparent and without color. There should be no white blood cells in the spinal fluid; however, a cell count of up to 10 is still considered normal by many physicians. Normally the fluid contains 5 to 15 mg per 100 ml of protein, 45 to 80 mg per 100 ml of sugar, and 110 to 125 mEq per liter of chloride.

Abnormal values: The spinal fluid pressure may be lower than normal when there is a spinal cord tumor or shock, or even after fainting. In diabetic coma the pressure is decreased. The pressure is increased following brain and spinal cord injury and in infection.

The color may have a reddish tinge if there is bleeding into the spinal canal following injury or stroke. With infection or with old blood from previous damage, the color may change to yellow or gray.

The cell count rises with infection, tumor, and most conditions that directly affect the brain, spinal cord, and their coverings.

Chemical tests for sugar and chloride are used to differentiate poliomyelitis from meningitis. Protein is elevated in almost all diseases that are reflected in the spinal fluid.

CEREBROSPINAL FLUID SCAN, see *Nuclear Scanning*

CERULOPLASMIN, see *Copper*

CERVICAL VISCOSITY, see *Tackmeter*

CERVIX, see *Schiller*

CHILDREN'S APPERCEPTION (CAT), see *Thematic Apperception*

CHLORIDE

Chloride, a salt of hydrochloric acid, is usually taken into the body as part of salt (sodium chloride). It is usually tested along with **Bicarbonate**, **Potassium**, and **Sodium**, since they all act reciprocally to balance the body's acid-base system and control water metabolism. The major concentration of chloride is in the tissues around cells and in stomach secretions (a very dilute hydrochloric acid). The kidney usually excretes about as much chloride as is taken in. Blood is collected from a vein and the serum is examined. Urine and spinal fluid may also be examined for chloride content.

When performed: When dizziness, weakness, or unconsciousness cannot easily be diagnosed; when adrenal disease is suspected.

Normal values: Normal values in the serum range from 100 to 110 mEq per liter (350 to 385 mg per 100 ml); in the urine, from 100 to 250 mEq per 24-hour sample; in the spinal fluid, from 120 to 130 mEq per liter.

Abnormal values: Serum chloride levels are occasionally elevated with kidney disease (but can be normal), dehydration, and aspirin toxicity. They are decreased with vomiting, diarrhea, excessive sweating, diuresis (with or without drugs), heart disease, and diabetic acidosis. Spinal fluid levels are usually decreased with meningitis; urine levels are decreased with hypoactive adrenal disease.

A special test called Robinson-Power-Kepler is used occasionally to help diagnose Addison's disease (inadequate adrenal function). After drinking a great deal of water, patients with the disease excrete higher than normal amounts of chloride in the urine but lower than normal amounts of water.

CHOLANGIOGRAPHY, see *Radiography*

CHOLECYSTOGRAPHY, see *Radiography*

CHOLESTEROL

Cholesterol is an essential body product that is manufactured by many organs such as the liver, the skin, and the intestines. It is not a fat, as is erroneously believed, but is a solid alcohol called a steroid; steroid compounds also include hormones, vitamins, and drugs. It has been estimated that the average person ingests about 600 mg of cholesterol each day. Cholesterol is found in most foods of animal origin; plant foods are usually free of the substance. Some representative examples of foods that contain cholesterol and the approximate amounts include:

a 4 ounce portion of brains	500 mg
a 4 ounce portion of liver, sweetbreads, or kidney	350 mg
a whole large size egg (or just the yolk)	250 mg
4 ounces of beef, pork, lamb, chicken or fish	80 mg
an 8 ounce glass of whole milk	25 mg

Cholesterol is indispensable for brain and nervous system growth and development (nerves cannot transmit impulses without it) as well as for the body's manufacture of sex hormones.

Cholesterol measurements are not very specific for diagnosing disease, and for many years the test was virtually abandoned; recently it has had a resurgence as a possible predictor of heart problems. Its actual predictive value has not yet been proved, however, and it is not totally accepted as a reliable heart risk measurement by most scientists and many cardiologists. Cardiac surgeons, who usually treat the most severe heart and artery disease, report that 80% of their patients have normal blood cholesterol levels.

The usual laboratory test measures total cholesterol, or all the cholesterol that is attached to various fats and proteins floating in the blood. However, when it comes to studying heart disease prediction, the specific protein-fat complexes (see **Lipoproteins**) to which the cholesterol is attached are more important. An excess of certain cholesterols—called alpha, or high-density lipoprotein (HDL) cholesterols—is associated with a *decrease* in heart disease. When cholesterol combines with a fatty acid, it is called a cholesterol ester.

Blood cholesterol levels will rise almost instantaneously when an individual is frightened, under anxiety, or in pain, and even when an individual is exposed to an uncomfortably loud noise. For example, many income tax accountants have a great increase in their cholesterol levels during the weeks before April 15; the elevated levels return to normal by May 1. Blood is taken from a vein and the serum is examined.

When performed: When there is suspicion of thyroid disease; with liver disease when there is a question of drug damage or hepatitis; with people who have xanthomatosis (yellowish plaques around the eyes, on the eyelids, over the elbows, and on the palms), although more than half of all people with xanthomatosis have normal cholesterol values; to measure the body's reaction to adrenal hormones; to measure an individual's response to stressful situations; as an experimental aid in the prediction of heart disease.

Normal values: Normal serum cholesterol levels range from 150 to 280 mg per 100 ml. These figures are not absolute. Higher values are normally found in older people; and with patients over 50 years of age, most laboratories consider 350 mg the upper limit of normal. Normal values also vary with the technique used (automated testing is considered less accurate and produces higher values).

Abnormal values: Serum cholesterol is increased with familial hypercholesteremia (an inherited trait); with hypothyroidism (cretinism), hepatitis, and kidney disease (nephrosis); and when the flow of bile from the gall bladder is obstructed. Elevated cholesterol levels also result from pregnancy (after the second month); from fear of the test results at the time the test is performed; and from taking male hormones, certain tranquilizers, cortisone products, vitamins A and D, some diuretic drugs, and epinephrine (adrenalin) products such as those used by asthmatics. Eating a great deal of cholesterol within a few hours of the test may have a slight effect on some people, but it is not constant.

Lower than normal cholesterol values are usually found with hyperthyroidism (Graves' disease), cirrhosis of the liver, certain anemias, and severe infections. Taking female hormones, thyroid hormones, aspirin, vitamin C or B_3 (niacin), certain antibiotics, and drugs used to treat diabetes will lower cholesterol values.

Decreased cholesterol esters indicate liver disease (hepatitis or active cirrhosis).

CHOLINESTERASE

There are two different forms of cholinesterase: one may be referred to as true cholinesterase, or acetylcholinesterase, and the other as pseudo-cholinesterase. Both enzymes are necessary for proper functioning of the parasympathetic nervous system, which controls the body's involuntary processes that transmit nerve impulses to the heart, gastrointestinal tract, tear ducts, etc. When these processes are reduced or interfered with—either by disease or by inhalation, ingestion, or skin contact with organic phosphate insecticide such as malathion—the patient has increased parasympathetic nervous system activity. Symptoms include increased stomach acidity, increased intestinal motility, erratic pulse and heart rate, difficulty in breathing, increased sweating, salivation, and watering of the eyes.

In almost all instances, pinpoint-sized pupils are an early sign of interference with the parasympathetic nervous system. Severe reactions include headache, muscle twitching, convulsions, and diarrhea. Some physicians believe ingestion of monosodium glutamate can also cause these reactions. True cholinesterase is measured from red blood cells; pseudo-cholinesterase is measured from serum. Both are obtained from blood taken from a patient's vein.

A special test to measure the presence of cholinesterase is the succinylcholine reaction. Succinylcholine is administered, and if cholinesterase is missing the patient will experience severe difficulty in breathing and muscle inactivity. The test is sometimes given by an anesthetist just prior to surgery to make sure that cholinesterase is present. Succinylcholine may also be used to aid in relaxation during surgery.

When performed: When a variety of symptoms that result from excessive parasympathetic nervous system activity are observed (as described above), especially after possible exposure to an insecticide; in certain skin, liver, and kidney diseases.

Normal values: Cholinesterase values in serum average at least 0.5 pH units per hour. In red blood cells true cholinesterase levels should be at least 0.7 pH units per hour. Some laboratories report cholinesterase values in their own units; these may range from 40 to 80 units as a total value.

Abnormal values: Decreased values indicate interference with the enzyme, usually as a result of organic phosphate poisoning. (Some physicians believe that the lower the value, the greater the intensity of the phosphate poisoning.) Cholinesterase may also be decreased during pregnancy and with cancer, liver disease, and certain skin conditions. Rarely, the levels are increased in kidney disease and hyperthyroidism.

CHORIONIC GONADOTROPIN, see *Pregnancy*; *Testis Function*

CHRISTMAS TREE, see *White Blood Cell*

CHROMATIN

All normal body cells have 46 chromosomes, including a set of sex chromosomes called chromatin cells. In the chromatin test the inside of the cheek is scraped for a minute specimen (called a buccal smear), and the cells are stained and examined under the microscope; these cells will reveal the presence or absence of a particular active sexual identity cell called the Barr body. The normal female cell has one Barr body and no Y-chromatin. The normal male cell shows no Barr body and one Y-chromatin. (The **Amniocentesis** test is a more detailed study of the chromosome makeup of the unborn infant.) White blood cells from venous blood may also be used in chromatin testing. Buccal smears are used primarily for screening to determine genetic sex; additional tests with the white blood cells are required for definitive information.

When performed: Whenever there is some doubt about the gender of the individual; whenever abnormal sexual development seems evident—either mentally or physically (undescended testicles, abnormal hair distribution, abnormal fat distribution, growth problems, infertility, failure to menstruate, and gynecomastia, or large breasts in a male).

Normal values: There should be no Barr body in the male and one Barr body in the female. Each cell should contain exactly 46 chromosomes.

Abnormal values: Abnormal values include finding only 45 chromosomes with no Barr body and finding 47 or more chromosomes with one or more Barr bodies. Most of these conditions produce physical sexual developmental abnormalities that usually become obvious with growth.

CHROMOSOME ANALYSIS, see *Amniocentesis*

CIA, see *Macroglobulin*

CINEANGIOGRAPHY, see *Radarkymogram*

CINERADIOGRAPHY, see *Radiography*

CIRCULATION TIME

The circulation time test determines just how fast the blood travels through the body. Usually a substance with a distinctive taste (saccharin, magnesium sulfate, or Epsom salts) is injected into an arm vein, and the exact time from the injection to the moment the patient "tastes" the substance (indicating its arrival at the tongue) is noted. The test may also be performed with dyes or with radioactive substances that are detected by nuclear scanners. The circulation time is affected by the amount of blood in the arteries and veins, especially by the speed with which the blood passes through the heart and lungs.

When performed: Primarily as an index of heart failure and its degree; sometimes as a measure of the circulation through the lungs, when the heart is known to be normal.

Normal values: In the "taste" test it should take from 8 to 16 seconds for the drug to go from the arm vein to the heart, through the lungs, back to the heart, and then into the arteries, particularly the arteries of the tongue, when the patient will taste the drug. Dye and radioactive tests take less time.

Abnormal values: Failure to "taste" the drug within 20 seconds is usually indicative of heart failure.

CISTERNOGRAPHY, see *Nuclear Scanning*

CLOTTING TIME, see *Bleeding and Clotting Time*

CO2, see *Carbon Dioxide*

COAGULATION TIME, see *Bleeding and Clotting Time*

COAGULOMETER

Because the drug heparin is being used more and more not only for the treatment of clotting disease but also for the prevention of blood clots, a new, simple test has been devised to measure the activity of this anticoagulant drug. Unlike the **Partial Thromboplastin Time** test, which requires venous blood, the coagulometer test can be performed with a blood sample from the fingertip and is similar to the **Bleeding and Clotting Time** tests. The blood is placed in the coagulometer tube, which is immersed in a solution at body temperature.

Because the coagulometer is a relatively new device, the test results are often compared with the partial thromboplastin time at regular intervals. The coagulometer test is especially valuable in controlling the dosage of heparin.

When performed: Before patients undergo surgery, especially surgery that will require a prolonged inactive convalescence (such as hip operations); when patients are being treated with low-dose heparin injections for thromboembolism.

Normal values: Blood in the special coagulometer tube usually clots within 1 to 2 minutes.

Abnormal values: If blood in the coagulometer tube clots sooner than 1 minute, this is considered a sign that the patient is prone to develop thrombosis. If the blood takes longer than 2.5 minutes to clot, this indicates that the patient has had too much heparin or has a tendency to bleed easily.

COBALAMINE, see *Schilling*

COCCIDIOIDOMYCOSIS, see *Complement Fixation*

COGNITIVE CAPACITY SCREENING

The cognitive capacity screening test aids in making one of the most difficult of all diagnoses: whether ostensible mental illness is organic (caused by brain damage or metabolic problems) or functional (caused by an inability or unwillingness to behave properly). Conventional mental status examinations (simply talking with a patient) may miss mental problems caused by physical disease.

In the cognitive capacity screening test, the patient is asked 30 questions. (For example: "Listen to these numbers—8, 1, 4, 3. Now count from 1 to 10 out loud and then repeat 8, 1, 4, 3." "Take 7 away from 100 and what do you have? Now take 7 away from that answer and keep taking 7 away from each answer.")

This test is becoming more and more important because of the increasing nursing-home population. Some institutions (as well as some public and private mental hospitals) tend to medicate their patients with tranquilizers and antidepressant drugs before determining if the patient's behavior has an organic or psychological basis. Such drugs will make true dementia cases seem much worse than they really are.

When performed: To ascertain a patient's ability to think, reason, and remember; to distinguish between organic dementia and functional delirium; to help diagnose brain pathology.

Normal values: Answering 20 or more questions correctly usually indicates no organic mental disease.

Abnormal values: Fewer than 20 correct answers should cause further investigation into the possibility of brain disease. Answering more than 20 questions correctly and still acting in a bizarre fashion usually indicates a psychotic reaction. Loss of memory for recent events with clear recall of incidents long past is another indication of many forms of dementia, especially Alzheimer's disease (senile dementia).

COLD AGGLUTINATION, see *Agglutination*

COLD CALORIC, see *Caloric*

COLD SORE, see *Herpes*

COLONOSCOPY, see *Endoscopy*

COLON X-RAY, see *Radiography*

COLOR BLINDNESS

About one in every 25 men (and one in every 250 women) cannot perceive the difference between red and green. This condition is almost always inherited. Very rarely, people cannot tell the difference between blue and yellow. The color blindness test usually consists of a special color plate made up of various colored dots that form numbers or figures. For example, a triangle or number 7 in red, orange, and yellow dots may be surrounded by many blue, green, and violet dots. The plate is shown to the patient, who is asked to describe the numbers or shapes.

Several different tests of color blindness (Ishihara, Hardy-Rand Rittler, HRR) are used, since people sometimes memorize a particular test in order to pass. Various colored lamps may also be used to detect those who either pretend to be color blind or who try to hide the condition.

When performed: On people whose occupation requires color discrimination (pilots, truck drivers, etc.).

Normal values: No matter how many different colored dots make up a color plate, a normal individual can distinguish the number or figures imprinted within a design of other colors.

Abnormal values: Someone who is color blind will be unable to discriminate a specific number or object among the many colored dots. Color blindness may be a consequence of alcoholism with blue-yellow defects being the most common.

COMPATIBLE TRANSFUSION, see *Typing and Cross-Matching*

COMPLEMENT

Serum complements are proteins in the blood that are part of the antigen-antibody system, which both fights and sometimes causes autoimmune disease (see **Agglutination**; **Antinuclear Antibodies**). There are at least 15 different forms of complement known at the present time; they are usually tested for as total complement, but they can be measured individually. Some forms of complement help neutralize viruses and destroy bacteria; others produce allergic reactions.

The complement decay rate test, also called the complement-1 esterase inhibitor test, is specific for diagnosing hereditary angioneurotic edema (a condition in which the skin, mucous membranes, and body organs, especially the lungs, suddenly swell up and become red). Blood is taken from a vein and the complement is measured from serum.

When performed: To differentiate familial angioneurotic edema from the noninherited allergic form of the disease (a far less serious condition); whenever autoimmune disease such as lupus erythematosus or scleroderma is suspected; in undiagnosed arthritis and kidney disease; when there is an overwhelming infection without a known cause.

Normal values: Total complement ranges from 50 to 100 CH_{50} units per ml. Normal values may vary with the method used. Normal values for individual components of complement (such as C-1, C-2, C-3) vary too widely with each laboratory to list any standard; the reported value is really a relative increase or decrease in the total complement and each component.

Abnormal values: Increased amounts of total complement are found with infections, jaundice, gout, after heart attacks, and sometimes with rheumatoid arthritis. Increased C-3 is found with cancer. Decreased amounts of complement (which are of greater significance) are found in a great many conditions, including chronic kidney disease, severe liver disease, lupus erythematosus, serum sickness (a severe allergic reaction), and myasthenia gravis.

COMPLEMENT FIXATION

The complement fixation test, which aids in the diagnosis of many diseases, relies on forms of serum antibody proteins (called **Complement**) being present in the blood to identify the specific disease under consideration. Antibodies are formed when the body is exposed to infections; if the antigens (specific causes) of the disease are mixed with a patient's serum, along with specially prepared sheep red blood cells, the antibodies and the antigens will combine and the blood cells will remain whole. If, on the other hand, the patient's serum does not contain complement antibodies to the disease, the sheep red blood cells will dissolve (a process called hemolysis).

Blood is taken from a vein and the serum is tested. The serum is diluted to the lowest concentration (highest dilution) that will give a positive reaction (no hemolysis) and is reported as that dilution, called titer. The test is related to the **Agglutination** reaction test, except that agglutination depends on the clumping together of the red blood cells as opposed to their staying whole and separate or their destruction. (At times the same disease will give a positive reaction to both the complement fixation test and the agglutination test.)

The precipitin reaction is another form of complement fixation test. It is particularly valuable in diagnosing suspected fungus diseases, especially aspergillosis of the lung (an infection that usually accompanies and aggravates asthma).

When performed: The test is used most often when there is suspicion of a virus-caused disease that cannot be accurately diagnosed. A few bacterial and fungus diseases also show a positive complement fixation test. Some specific diseases that can yield a positive high-dilution complement fixation include:

Blastomycosis (a fungus-caused lung disease)

Coccidioidomycosis (a fungus-caused disease that begins in the lung, sometimes called valley fever)

Dengue fever (breakbone fever)

Encephalitis (also to differentiate the kind)
Gastroenteritis
Gonorrhea
Hemorrhagic fever
Hydatid disease (echinococcosis)
Influenza (also to distinguish types A, B, and C)
Lassa fever (a new African disease)
Meningitis (primarily virus-caused)
Pneumonia (primarily virus-caused)
Poliomyelitis
Psittacosis (a pneumonia-type disease from bird droppings)
Syphilis
Tick fever
Tuberculosis
Venereal diseases

Normal values: Because of possible past unknown or unremembered infections, an unchanging low-titer positive reaction (a reaction in a very strong or slightly diluted solution) to many diseases is not considered unusual.

Abnormal values: A high titer (a reaction in a very weak or highly diluted solution) to a suspected disease, especially a titer that rises even higher (becomes positive in more highly diluted solutions of serum) after a week or two, indicates the presence of disease. Although the test is used mostly to diagnose suspected disease, it can also be positive in cases of thyroid infection, gout, and severe allergic conditions. Some of the 15 different forms of Complement may be reduced in a variety of diseases, usually of the inherited type, but also with various forms of arthritis, certain anemias, malaria, and systemic lupus erythematosus.

COMPLETE BLOOD COUNT, see *Blood Cell Differential*; *Red Blood Cell*; *White Blood Cell*

COMPUTERIZED TOMOGRAPHY (CT, CAT)

Tomography (see **Radiography**) is the focusing of X-rays on a specific level or plane of the body (as if one passed a thin piece of photographic paper through, say, the abdomen, and recorded only what was in that layer of tissue that the film touched). All other areas above, below, or to either side of that plane are obliterated. With computerized tomography (CT), the extremely narrow X-ray beam passes through a cross section of the body (or the brain) and is picked up by an electronic instrument called a scintillator rather than being exposed on the usual X-ray film. The scintillator then feeds into a computer exactly what density (thickness or thinness) of tissue the X-rays passed through. The computer prints out the densities as an illustration of that cross section of the body. Bone, which is of the highest density, comes out white in the picture. Liquids and air, which are of the lowest density, come out black. In between are all shades of gray representing various organs and tissues.

Unlike the typical X-ray exposure, the X-ray camera and scintillator rotate extremely rapidly around the body section being photographed so as to include everything in equal focus. CT is sometimes referred to as transaxial tomography or computerized axial tomography (CAT) because it represents a cross section of the long axis (standing-erect position) of the body. To perform CT on the entire head or a particular body section such as the chest or abdomen takes only one second, and the total amount of X-ray exposure is far less than one old-fashioned X-ray picture. CT images may be viewed on a television screen or reproduced as photographs for permanent study.

There are two different forms of CT: brain scanning and whole-body scanning. CT scanning is different from **Nuclear Scanning** in that no radioactive chemicals are injected into the body. The machines used for each type of scanning are slightly different. Both types of scanning require that the patient remain absolutely motionless for accurate results.

There has been some controversy over CT scanning within the medical profession and especially within the insurance industry, which must pay the costs of the tests. CT scanning is relatively expensive compared with other techniques such as regular X-ray. Furthermore, only a few physicians can be considered experts in the field, since the device was first used in 1973. At the same time, costly as these new machines are, they have been shown to eliminate the need for a great deal of "exploratory" surgery (operations simply to help diagnose a disease, not to cure it). CT scans have also demonstrated that certain allegedly therapeutic surgery would be ineffective if performed. There is general agreement that CT scanning can eliminate potentially dangerous and not always rewarding tests, such as pneumoencephalograms and arteriography (see **Radiography**).

Positron emission transaxial tomography (**PETT**) is similar to CT, but utilizes radiolabeled substances such as glucose to measure some body functions (metabolic rates in different regions of the body that show the effect of treatment in diseases such as stroke).

When performed: The test is performed whenever brain pathology is suspected, especially brain substance deterioration (dementia), as well as after any head injury, especially to detect a subdural hematoma (although this may not show up on a CT scan for several days). It is also used when brain tumors are suspected; sometimes a contrast dye is injected into a neck artery so that the dye will more clearly demarcate the lesion. CT scanning may be used when hydrocephalus (or any increase in cerebrospinal fluid pressure) is suspected.

Body scanning is performed primarily when there are abdominal or chest problems that cannot be diagnosed by the usual tests. A CT cross section can illustrate the size and shape of all the body organs and their relationship to adjacent organs and tissues. Such a test is especially valuable when pancreatic pathology is suspected (tumors, cysts, hemorrhage, edema) and when liver disease is being considered, especially problems with the bile ducts. It is also valuable in detecting kidney masses and how well the kidneys are functioning, particularly when there is suspected disease of the retroperitoneal space between the abdominal organs and the back muscles and spine (abscesses, hematomas, tumors, diseases of the great blood vessels such as the aorta and large abdominal veins, and lymph node and lymph channel blockage).

Abdominal CT scanning has proved especially valuable when a patient has stomach pains and no evident cause can be found. Many doctors now feel that chest and lung diseases that were once very difficult to diagnose (conditions such as sarcoidosis; old, hidden tuberculosis; enlarged arteries and veins) can be detected by body scanning.

Diseases of the extremities (especially bone and muscle) are being diagnosed by CT more and more often as experience lends itself to greater expertise.

Normal values: A CT scan should show no abnormality in the size and position of organs and tissues.

Abnormal values: Only with extensive experience are doctors able to interpret abnormal findings in a CT illustration and then make a specific diagnosis from that finding. For example, when there is evidence of dementia or physical brain disease, a brain scan will show the convolutions between the brain folds to be much wider than normal—something that cannot be detected by any other test. When CT scans are taken at different levels of the brain, the extent of the disease (along with the possibility of successful treatment) can sometimes be determined. In body scanning, an experienced physician can detect minute pathology such as cysts and tumors that would not be revealed by other tests.

CONGO RED

Congo red is a dye used in testing for amyloidosis (a disease condition in which amyloid, a compound mixture of proteins resembling starch, is deposited in various parts of the body, usually in the connective tissue spaces between body cells). Many physicians feel amyloidosis is an abnormality of the plasma cells that produce immunoglobulins and thus is similar to multiple myeloma (see **Bence-Jones Protein**). The Congo red test is not performed as frequently as it was in the past; today the diagnosis of amyloidosis is usually made from a **Biopsy** of amyloid-looking tissue. The test is still utilized when a patient has a generalized total-body-reaction disease of a mysterious nature.

The patient is asked to fast for 12 hours before the test. Congo red dye is injected intravenously; two minutes later the first of two specimens is withdrawn from a vein for examination of the serum. One hour later a second blood sample is taken and the serum is tested for the amount of dye still present. The urine is also tested.

When performed: When amyloidosis is suspected; when there is unexplained weight loss, or small hemorrhages of the skin; when kidney disease is suspected.

Normal values: After one hour the serum should still contain at least 60% of the Congo red dye. The urine should show no dye.

Abnormal values: In systemic amyloidosis (where the entire body is involved), almost all the dye leaves the serum and is absorbed by the amyloid tissue; from 0 to 10% may be recovered after an hour. With kidney amyloidosis, the serum will show about 40% of the dye, and the urine will contain large amounts.

CONTACT LENS, see *Fluorescein Eye Stain*

CONTRACEPTION, see *Body Temperature*

CONTRAST RADIOGRAPHY, see *Radiography*

COOMBS', see *Agglutination*

COORDINATION, see *Cerebellum*

COPPER

Copper is an essential nutrient. The body requires approximately 2 to 5 mg of copper a day. There are many dietary sources of copper (liver, oysters, beans, peas, avocado, whole grains), so deficiency is relatively uncommon. Copper is measured in the blood serum. In the body copper combines with the protein ceruloplasmin, which can also be measured in the serum as an indication of copper content. Copper is sometimes measured in the urine and in hair (the latter measure is quite reliable).

When performed: When there is suspicion of Wilson's disease (heptolenticular or liver degeneration); in anemia and pregnancy; in patients taking oral contraceptives.

Normal values: Normal serum copper levels range from 75 to 150 mcg per 100 ml. Normal ceruloplasmin levels range from 20 to 45 mg per 100 ml or 35 to 65 IU. Normal urine levels of copper range from 15 to 40 mcg in a 24-hour sample.

Abnormal values: Serum copper levels may be increased in cirrhosis of the liver, leukemia, pregnancy, anemia, heart attack, and infections. Decreased serum copper levels are found in Wilson's disease and sprue. Increased ceruloplasmin is seen in pregnancy, heart attack, infections, cirrhosis of the liver, and patients taking oral contraceptives. Decreased ceruloplasmin is found with kwashiorkor disease and Wilson's disease and in infants with anemia and hypoproteinemia.

COPROPORPHYRIN, see *Lead*; *Porphyrins*

CORNEAL REFLEX, see *Reflex*

CORNEAL STAINING, see *Fluorescein Eye Stain*

CORNELL INDEX

The Cornell Medical Index Health Questionnaire is a medical history test that the patient fills out at home before his first interview with the physician. In the section related to bodily symptoms, the questionnaire covers eyes, ears, respiratory system, cardiovascular system, digestive tract, musculoskeletal system, skin, nervous system, genitourinary system, fatigability, frequency of illness, and habits. There are also questions about family history, past illnesses, and moods and feelings (depression, anxiety, sensitivity, inadequacy, anger, tension).

When performed: The index is used as a preliminary test to aid in diagnosis of the individual patient as well as in mass screening. It is especially valuable in distinguishing between psychological and physical problems.

Normal values: Interpretations are based largely on the physician's assessment, which includes an interview with the patient and a physical examination along with the Cornell Medical Index. In general, there should be fewer than 25 "yes" answers.

Abnormal values: The "yes" answers form a pattern that indicates the patient's medical as well as psychological problem areas. More than 25 "yes" answers indicate a serious problem; answering both "yes" and "no" to the same question, omitting answers on six or more questions, or adding remarks to three questions or more are all considered indicative of a problem.

CORONARY ANGIOGRAPHY, see *Radiography*

CORONARY HEART DISEASE RISK, see *Jenkins Activity Survey*

CORTICOSTEROIDS, see *Cortisol*

CORTISOL

Cortisol (hydrocortisone) is manufactured from cholesterol. It is the main glucocorticoid hormone (a hormone with anti-inflammatory and metabolic activity) secreted by the cortex (outside layers) of the adrenal glands. Cortisol not only reduces the body's protective reactions to bacteria; it also acts on blood sugar levels by inhibiting insulin, helps control protein metabolism, redistributes fat in the body from the arms and legs to the torso, and regulates body water distribution by directing the excretion of sodium and potassium. The amount of cortisol secreted by the cortex is controlled (1) by the hypothalamus portion of the brain, which reacts to physical and emotional stress as well as to other observations of the senses such as noise, odors, and light and darkness; (2) by the pituitary gland, which reacts to how much cortisol is in the blood; and (3) as a consequence of any abnormalities within the adrenal glands (such as tumors).

The adrenal glands normally produce the greatest amount of cortisol in the early morning and the smallest amount in the evening. When a person's regular hours are changed (as by working nights and sleeping days), the cortisol secretion rates are usually reversed. Thus, when testing for cortisol, it is vital to know the patient's active and sleeping times. It is also important to know the mental state of the patient, since emotions have a strong influence on the adrenal glands. Blood is collected from a vein and the plasma is tested. Urine is also regularly tested.

When adrenal disease is considered, it is usual to perform an adrenal suppression test. A synthetic glucocorticoid drug such as dexamethasone is given to the patient, and cortisol levels are measured for several days afterward. A patient with normal adrenal glands will show a marked reduction in cortisol secretion the next day and for as long as the drug is administered. With Cushing's syndrome, the adrenal suppression test shows that the adrenals do not stop secreting cortisol; and if cortisol is not even slightly reduced after the first two days, an adrenal tumor is usually indicated. An opposite approach, called the ACTH stimulation test, while not as accurate, may also be employed. ACTH (the pituitary hormone that causes the adrenals to secrete cortisol) is injected. If there is no increase in plasma cortisol, an adrenal tumor is indicated.

In the metyrapone test the patient is given the drug metyrapone, which prevents direct cortisol production, in order to determine if ACTH will stimulate the adrenals. The drug is usually given at midnight and cortisol levels are measured the next morning. Normally the drug-induced reduction in cortisol will cause the body's ACTH to stimulate cortisol production; failure to produce cortisol indicates that the problem lies within the pituitary gland rather than in the adrenals. In patients taking birth control pills or other estrogens, this test can be falsely positive. On rare occasions insulin is given to provoke cortisol secretions; a normal response is a large rise in plasma cortisol.

There are several other tests to measure adrenal cortex function. Two that are used frequently are the urinary 17-ketosteroids (17-KS) and the urinary 17-hydroxycorticosteroids. The latter measures how much cortisol the adrenals are secreting. The former (17-KS), once the most common adrenal test performed, is no longer considered the most reliable measurement of adrenal activity.

When performed: The test is used primarily to diagnose adrenocortical function such as when Cushing's syndrome (excessive adrenal activity) or Addison's disease (inflammation of the adrenals) is suspected. It is also used when there is precocious puberty, hirsutism (excessive body hair), and excessive signs of feminization in men.

Normal values: Normal cortisol values in plasma are less than 30 mcg per 100 ml in the morning and less than 10 mcg per 100 ml in the evening. There should be no more than 10 mcg per 100 ml in a 24-hour urine sample.

Abnormal values: Plasma cortisol levels are increased in stress. In Cushing's syndrome normal night and day variations in cortisol levels are lacking. Cortisol levels are reduced with Addison's disease and with excessive androgenic (masculinizing) hormone activity. Urine levels are increased with Cushing's syndrome and with hyperthyroidism and obesity.

COUMARIN, see *Prothrombin Time*

COVER-UNCOVER, see *Strabismus*

C-PEPTIDE

C-peptide (the C stands for "connecting") is a portion of the basic material used by the body to manufacture insulin. The test, employed primarily in patients with diabetes, measures how much (if any) insulin the patient's pancreas can manufacture. Commercial insulin contains no C-peptide; thus a patient taking regular injections of insulin can still be tested to find out if he is producing any insulin of his own. Knowing if a patient is producing natural insulin (even in small amounts) affects the type of treatment for diabetes. Most often urine is tested; blood serum from a vein may also be measured for C-peptide.

When performed: The test is performed at regular intervals whenever diabetes is known or suspected to ascertain body insulin capability. It is also used to detect if a patient is taking erroneous (usually excessive) doses of insulin and to verify suspected hypoglycemia (low blood sugar). Urine testing is preferred with children when blood specimens are difficult to obtain.

Normal values: There are no specific numerical values for C-peptide. Its presence indicates that the body can manufacture insulin; its absence indicates that there is no insulin production.

Abnormal values: Failure to detect C-peptide after giving a patient glucose to stimulate insulin production usually indicates diabetes. Lack of C-peptide in the blood can also mean that a patient has taken so much insulin that the pancreas has shut down because it has no need to produce the hormone. Large amounts of C-peptide can indicate overactive insulin-producing cells in the pancreas, which can cause hypoglycemia.

CPK, see *Creatine Phosphokinase*

C-REACTIVE PROTEIN (CRP)

C-reactive protein (CRP) is a blood gamma globulin that reacts with certain bacterial substances in many inflammatory conditions. The CRP test is not specific for any one disease. At one time the test was in widespread use in diagnosing and following patients with rheumatic fever; today the erythrocyte **Sedimentation Rate** (ESR), a similar but simpler and less expensive test, is often used in place of the CRP. Blood is taken from a vein and the serum is tested. In a few disease conditions, especially rheumatic fever, CRP may show up in blood serum before the ESR is elevated.

When performed: In conditions causing inflammation and tissue breakdown; to note progress in the treatment of certain illnesses such as rheumatoid arthritis, tuberculosis, and viral infections.

Normal values: C-reactive proteins are not normally found in the blood.

Abnormal values: C-reactive proteins are found in measurable amounts with bacterial and viral infections, rheumatic fever, cancer, arthritis, heart attack, and pneumonia. Aspirin or steroid drugs will mask the appearance of CRP.

CREATINE, see *Creatinine*

CREATINE PHOSPHOKINASE (CPK)

Creatine phosphokinase (CPK) is an enzyme that is found predominantly in skeletal muscle, heart muscle, and the brain. When muscle is damaged, CPK leaks out into the bloodstream. When heart muscle is damaged, most commonly after a heart attack, CPK blood serum levels will rise within hours after the attack. Of all the different enzymes that are usually liberated when heart muscle is damaged, CPK is increased most rapidly (within six hours). It is believed that the rise in CPK is proportionate to the amount of damaged heart muscle.

When performed: To verify suspected heart attack; to ascertain muscular disease and to follow the progress of illness; to help discover genetic carriers of progressive muscular dystrophy; to distinguish malignant hyperthermia (abnormally high fever after receiving certain anesthetics) from fever due to postoperative infection.

Normal values: CPK values can vary with different laboratories. Generally, up to 12 Sigma units and up to 50 IU are considered normal.

Abnormal values: CPK levels are almost always elevated after a heart attack and with muscular dystrophy. Electrophoresis (separating the various forms of the enzyme with an electrical current) will usually distinguish between the two diseases. Hypothyroidism, alcoholism, and injury to the muscles (even intramuscular injections of medicines) can also cause increased CPK levels. Strenuous exercise can cause a very large increase in CPK, but this usually disappears after a day. With heart damage the CPK level takes three to four days to return to normal. Prolonged bed rest alone will lower CPK. Recently, increased CPK levels have been found in patients with asthma and other lung conditions that cause difficulty in breathing.

CREATININE

Creatinine is the end product of muscle metabolism (not from heart muscle, however). It is formed from creatine, which provides energy for the muscles to function. Both creatine and creatinine come from amino acids which result from the breakdown of dietary protein. Creatinine is often tested along with **Urea Nitrogen**, which is also primarily a measure of kidney function. (Creatinine is considered the better measure of the two.)

Virtually all creatinine is normally excreted by a part of the kidney called the glomerulus, which is the first of six different filter systems the kidney utilizes to retain products the body needs and to dispose of waste material. Although creatinine is frequently measured in blood serum, the most useful measurement is derived from urine.

The creatinine clearance test is performed on a specimen of urine collected over a 24-hour period. (A newer form of the creatinine clearance test requires the collection of urine only over a 5-hour period.) This test measures the glomerular filtration rate (normally about 5 ounces of blood are filtered by the kidneys each minute) and is thus a fairly reliable indicator of how well the kidneys are functioning.

The inulin clearance test is a bit more precise than creatinine clearance but much more difficult to perform. The urea clearance test is less reliable in that it is affected by diet and how much urine is passed. The PAH (sodium p-aminohippuric acid) clearance test is one of many new kidney function tests that work in a similar way to creatinine clearance. Creatine (not creatinine) is sometimes measured in the serum and the urine as a confirmation of creatinine clearance.

When performed: Primarily when there is suspicion of kidney damage; as an aid in the diagnosis of certain muscle diseases, especially those caused by hormone problems; when a liver problem cannot be specifically diagnosed.

Creatinine clearance is especially useful when there is an abnormal urea nitrogen test; the two tests together may help locate the specific area of kidney trouble. It also helps determine if a kidney problem is caused in part by bleeding or by the way protein in the diet affects the kidneys. The creatinine clearance test is of great value in determining the seriousness of kidney disease as well as in measuring the progress of treatment. It is also of special value when compared with the **Amylase** clearance test to diagnose pancreatitis.

Normal values: Blood serum creatinine values range from 0.8 to 1.3 mg per 100 ml. When measured in the urine, creatinine clearance is expressed as the glomerular filtration rate for a 24-hour period. For men, the normal range is between 110 and 170 ml per minute. Women usually have a slightly lower rate (90 ml per minute is still considered normal).

Abnormal values: Elevated serum creatinine along with reduced creatinine clearance indicates a kidney problem. The severity of the disease is indicated by the amount of reduced glomerular flow. When creatinine values are compared with urea nitrogen values, it is sometimes possible to ascertain if the kidney disease is reflecting the blood flow to the kidney or some blockage in the urinary tract between the kidney and the bladder. Serum creatinine is also increased in certain muscle diseases; when there is vomiting or diarrhea; when patients are taking certain drugs such as steroids, barbiturates, and vitamin C; and when large amounts of roast meats (which contain high levels of creatinine) are eaten.

CREMASTERIC, see *Reflex*

CROSS-EYES, see *Strabismus*

CROSS-MATCHING, see *Typing and Cross-Matching*

CRP, see *C-Reactive Protein*

CRYOGLOBULIN, see *Immunoglobulin*

CT, see *Computerized Tomography*

CULTURE

The purpose of a culture is to isolate and identify the microbes that cause disease by an infectious process. The science of microbiology (microbial culture) was formerly known as bacteriology. The name was changed after many organisms in addition to bacteria—viruses, fungi, rickettsia, parasites—were found to cause disease. Since virtually every part of the body is subject to infection, the test is performed on many tissues, secretions, excretions, and fluids. Blood, urine, spinal cord fluid, joint fluid, feces, bone marrow, and material from an abscess, ulcer, sinuses, eyes, ears, nose, and throat all may be cultured.

Some microbes do damage directly by their presence; others cause illness by giving off a toxic product (botulism toxin). Disease-causing microbes must always be distinguished from nonharmful organisms that normally live in various parts of the body. Thus, while a direct examination on a slide under a microscope may show bacteria, only a culture can positively identify the type of bacteria.

Usually a sample for culture is placed in two or more containers, each with a different medium (an environment that promotes growth)—one to grow organisms in the presence of air and one to grow them without air. Whenever the specimen is taken, absolute sterility must be observed to avoid contamination. If microbes grow in the sample, many other tests are performed to determine whether the microbes are pathological. Usually small bits of paper saturated with different antibiotic solutions are placed on the microbes to find out which drugs are most effective in killing them. This is called the antibiotic sensitivity test. Such testing is especially important today because so many microorganisms have become resistant to antibiotics.

When microbial infection is suspected, it is also common to perform **Agglutination** and **Complement Fixation** tests to confirm the identity of the organism. Viruses can now be cultured by using living cells (such as chick embryos in eggs) and then identified by agglutination, complement fixation, and electron microscope examination.

When performed: Whenever there are symptoms of infection (usually high fever) and no specific diagnosis can be made.

Normal values: There should be no growth of microorganisms from the various tissues, secretions, and body fluids (except for the normal bacteria in the intestines, throat, etc.).

Abnormal values: Any evident growth of pathological microorganisms is abnormal. When any disease-causing microorganisms are found in the blood, septicemia is indicated. Tuberculosis is diagnosed only by applying an acid-fast stain to distinguish the bacteria in the culture.

CUSHING'S SYNDROME, see *Cortisol*

CUTLER, see *Sedimentation Rate*

CYCLOPLEGIA, see *Visual Acuity*

CYSTIC FIBROSIS, see *Phytohemagglutinin*; *Sodium*

CYSTINURIA, see *Aminoaciduria*

CYSTOMETRY

Normally the bladder will hold about 12 ounces of fluid before the urge to urinate is felt. This urge is caused by the pressure of the fluid against the expanding bladder walls. When the exact response to bladder pressure must be determined, or when it is necessary to know if the patient can discriminate between warm and cold temperatures in the bladder, cystometry is performed.

A catheter (very thin tube) is inserted into the bladder through the urethra and attached to a manometer (a graduated glass tube showing the response to pressure measurements). The bladder is then filled, and the patient's response to known pressure (and the amount of fluid) is recorded. A Lewis cystometer produces a graph showing pressure and capacity response. When necessary, the bladder is then alternately filled with warm and cold water and the patient's response to varying temperatures is recorded.

When performed: Whenever a patient has difficulty urinating (voiding), especially when the patient lacks the normal urge to urinate (usually because of bladder nerve disease); with urinary infections; to test the effect of certain drugs on the bladder, especially when such drugs are to be used to extend the capacity of the bladder or to initiate a response in a bladder that overfills.

Normal values: Until the bladder contains almost a pint of fluid, there should be no uncomfortable sensations. Additional fluid normally causes discomfort, along with sweating and flushing, followed by the urge to urinate.

Abnormal values: Failure to feel pressure after 12 ounces of fluid are instilled in the bladder, along with the inability to distinguish between warm and cold solutions, usually indicates disease of the nerves to and from the spinal cord to the bladder. With infections, the bladder will feel full with only a small amount of fluid.

CYSTOSCOPY, see *Endoscopy*

CYTOLOGY

Cytology tests detect and identify both normal and abnormal cells (especially cancer cells) in areas that cannot be easily and directly examined. Specimens to be examined may be obtained from body excretions (urine, feces), secretions (sputum, gastric, eye, peritoneal, breast, prostatic, vaginal, and cerebrospinal fluid), and tissue scrapings (uterus, vagina, mouth, nose, throat, bronchi, rectum, stomach, and cysts). The test makes possible very early diagnosis and treatment of cancer. It can also indicate hormone activity in the body, as well as specific infections and the effect of radiation. After the smears are collected and stained, they are examined under a microscope. The unique tissue-staining technique used in the original test was devised by Dr. George Papanicolaou and is still called a Papanicolaou or Pap test by some doctors.

When performed: As a routine or screening test during a physical examination; whenever cancer is suspected; for hormonal assessment; when there is undiagnosed disease in a particular organ or body system.

Normal values: No abnormal cells should be seen in any stained smear.

Abnormal values: Any cancer cell or even a suspicious cell is considered a positive or abnormal result. A positive test is usually repeated. If the second test is still positive, a **Biopsy** (the removal of a minute piece of tissue from the suspected organ), X-rays (see **Radiography**), or other appropriate diagnostic tests must be performed to verify diagnosis. Inappropriate hormone influence on cells or evidence of inflammation is considered abnormal.

DAP, see *Pregnancy*

DARK FIELD, see *Syphilis*

D&C, see *Dilatation and Curettage*

DEEP REFLEX, see *Reflex*

DEEP-VEIN THROMBOSIS, see *Plethysmography*

DELTA AMINOLEVULINIC ACID (ALA), see *Lead*; *Porphyrins*

DEMENTIA, see *Cognitive Capacity Screening*

DEPRESSION

Depression is a mental state that can be caused by physical disease, after pregnancy, and with hormone changes, or it can be a personal reaction to an unpleasant situation. The usual symptoms of depression (tiredness, insomnia, lack of appetite, stomach and intestinal complaints, irritability) can mimic a great many other illnesses. Because of the close association between depression and suicide, it is important to diagnose true depression early.

There are several different questionnaire-type surveys that help to make the specific diagnosis of depression. In the Beck Depression Inventory, the patient is asked to select responses from several sets of leading statements. A set of statements may range, for example, from "I am dissatisfied with everything" to "I am not particularly dissatisfied." Proponents of this test claim that it aids not only in diagnosing depression but also in measuring the degree of depression.

A somewhat similar test is the Zung Self-Rating Depression Scale. The patient is asked to evaluate a series of self-descriptive statements such as "Morning is when I feel best" by checking off a column headed "none or a little of the time," "some of the time," " a good part of the time," or "most or all of the time." This test also claims to be able to indicate the degree of depression.

All such tests are really only screening devices; a positive diagnosis of depression must be based on in-depth doctor-patient interviews.

When performed: When patients have vague symptoms, especially tiredness, helplessness, or pessimistic feelings; after a stressful situation in a patient's life (loss of a loved one, loss of a job); when a patient is taking certain drugs, especially tranquilizers; when a patient has marital problems; when suicidal tendencies are suspected by the doctor.

Normal values: Most patients rarely select more than two or three statements that indicate depression.

Abnormal values: Four or more statements associated with a depressed state of mind can indicate mild depression; a greater number of such responses can indicate severe depression and potential suicide. Again, such tests should be used only as screening devices and should be followed by detailed interviews with the patient.

DEPTH PERCEPTION, see *Visual Acuity*

DERMATOME, see *Sensory Ability*

DIABETES MELLITUS, see *Glucose*

DIABETES MONITORING, see *Glycohemoglobin*

DIABETIC ACIDOSIS, see *Ketones*

DIAGNEX BLUE, see *Gastric Analysis*

DIAGNOSTIC CYTOLOGY, see *Cytology*

DIASTOLIC PRESSURE, see *Blood Pressure*

DICK, see *Skin Reaction*

DIFFERENTIAL, see *Blood Cell Differential*

DIFFUSING CAPACITY, see *Pulmonary Function*

DIGITALIS TOXICITY

Digitalis and its synthetic substitutes digoxin and digitoxin (called cardiac glycosides) are the most widely used drugs in congestive heart failure. They increase the force of the heartbeat and slow down the initiating impulse that causes the heart muscle to contract, decreasing the heart rate. Before digitalis, digoxin, or digitoxin is administered, it is essential to discover and follow in the patient the fine line between the amount of the drug necessary to achieve a therapeutic effect and the amount that will cause a toxic effect. Too much of one of these drugs can cause nausea, vomiting, and irregular heartbeats (which can be fatal).

The digitalis toxicity test measures the amount of digoxin or digitoxin in a patient's serum (whole-leaf digitalis is rarely used today). The patient should not take the drug for at least 8 to 12 hours prior to the test. Of equal importance, once a therapeutic dose has been established the patient must not change the brand of drug; it has been shown that different brands of the same drug at the same dose can be toxic because of different dissolving and absorption qualities.

When performed: To follow the course of therapy in patients taking digoxin, digitoxin, and other digitalis drugs in order to prevent poisoning.

Normal values: Normal values are those that produce a therapeutic effect without causing toxicity.

Abnormal values: Digoxin levels above 1.5 ng per ml are often found to be toxic; serum levels below 1.5 ng per ml are not usually toxic but are therapeutic. The therapeutic, nontoxic levels of digitoxin are usually less than 18 ng per ml. These figures are only examples; they vary widely for different individuals. For digoxin, up to 3.5 ng per ml has not been toxic, and for digitoxin up to 40 ng per ml has been safe. In other words, no two people have the same therapeutic, nontoxic blood level.

When digitalis toxicity tests are performed, it is important to test for **Potassium** (elevated serum potassium accentuates digitalis toxicity), **Calcium**, and **Creatinine** clearance (kidney function). Digoxin is excreted by the kidney; digitoxin through the liver; this is important if a patient has kidney or liver disease.

DIGITOXIN, see *Digitalis Toxicity*

DIGOXIN, see *Digitalis Toxicity*

DILANTIN, see *Drug Monitoring*

DILATATION AND CURETTAGE (D&C)

The D&C is perhaps the most frequently performed test in the diagnosis of gynecologic problems. The examination is usually performed in a hospital or a clinic under general anesthesia. For the dilatation part of the test, dilators of increasingly large circumference are used to create an opening large enough for examination of the cervical canal (the opening in the cervix to the uterus) and the endometrium (lining of the uterus). A curette (spoon-shaped instrument) is used to scrape the endometrial cavity (curettage) for tissue samples, which are then examined under a microscope. Endometrial screening may sometimes be performed by suction collection instead of scraping, and with this method it can be done in the physician's office, without anesthesia, using a jet irrigation and suction technique. (See **Endoscopy** for hysteroscopy following dilatation.)

When performed: When there is abnormal uterine bleeding or discharge; in infertility; in infections; when there is suspicion of anomaly (uterine abnormality); when there is suspicion of fibroids or cancer of the uterus or cervix; to ascertain the phase of the menstrual cycle; to remove polyps; for therapeutic abortion.

Normal values: Normally no malformations, blockage of the cervical canal, cancer cells, or polyps are found. The cells that line the uterus usually show hormone activity that conforms to menstrual cycle changes.

Abnormal values: Abnormal findings include tumor, cancerous cells, or cells in the uterine lining that do not match the expected phase of the menstrual cycle.

DINITROPHENYLHYDRAZINE, see *Phenylketonuria*

DIPHTHERIA, see *Skin Reaction*

DIPLOPIA, see *Strabismus*

DIRECT BILIRUBIN, see *Bilirubin*

DIRECT OPHTHALMOSCOPIC, see *Fundoscopy*

DISPUTED PARENTAGE

In all areas of the United States approximately 10% of all births are illegitimate; in some urban areas more than 50% of all newborn children are illegitimate. In light of recent court decisions giving the same legal rights to illegitimate children that legitimate children have (support, inheritance, and many other benefits), knowledge of parenthood has become important for legal reasons as well as for social reasons. There is the need to protect men who are falsely accused of fatherhood as well as to assure mothers that the children they bring home from the hospital are really theirs.

The term "paternity test" is a misnomer in that disputed parentage tests do not prove whether a man or woman is really the biological parent of a child; rather, they can only help prove that the man or woman *could not possibly be* the biological parent. At this time nearly 100 different tests can be performed, all of which point out that certain of the mother's or father's biological traits were or were not inherited by the child. Some are based on blood types (such as the O, A, B, AB, Rh, and hemoglobin groups); some are based on immunological characteristics that are transmitted from parent to child (such as enzyme defects, various globulin levels, and cell compatibility).

Sometimes only one test is needed to show that a child could not possibly be the issue of an alleged parent (for example, if an accused father has type AB blood and the child has type O blood). More often than not, however, seven basic tests are performed; it is claimed that these tests offer a probability of exclusion of 93%. After 62 different tests are performed, the probability of exclusion reaches 98%.

When such tests are performed today, an individual must have an instant-development photograph taken of his face and then affix his signature to the back of the photograph along with his thumbprint. This identifying material is attached to the report to show the specific individual on whom the tests were made. (In the past it was not unusual for a man to go to a laboratory, give the name of the accused father, and offer his blood for testing after earlier, private tests confirmed that the substitute man's blood would exclude him from parentage.) With children, photographs and footprints are used for identification. In addition, the tests are performed in two separate laboratories at the same time. Saliva may also be tested as a confirmatory measure, comparing inherited characteristics of the enzymes.

When performed: The test is used most often in legal disputes concerning births out of wedlock. The most common dispute involves a man accused of being the father of a child. In quite a few instances, however, a mother will claim that the child brought home from the hospital is not hers because of alleged child substitution.

Normal values: There are no normal values in disputed parentage tests since, even if all known tests show that a person could be the parent of a child, there is always a small margin of doubt. If, however, the tests show that parentage would be impossible, they are considered completely accurate. (For example, a woman with type A_2 blood could not possibly be the mother of a child whose blood type was A_1B, no matter who the father was.)

Abnormal values: The only possibility of error occurs when the laboratory's testing serum contains traces of other typing factors not noted on the label (this is not a rare occurrence).

DOLL'S EYE, see *Reflex*

DOPPLER, see *Ultrasound*

DOWN'S SYNDROME, see *Amniocentesis*

DRIVING UNDER THE INFLUENCE, see *Alcohol*

DRUG MONITORING

Most drugs that are prescribed are quite potent; the range of safety between the amount of a drug that is therapeutically effective and the amount that is toxic is very narrow. In addition, there are times when a prescribed drug seems to have no effect, either because of some idiosyncrasy in the patient's metabolism or because the patient is not taking the drug as prescribed. It is known that two out of three patients do not properly follow directions for a prescription drug, and one out of three patients never even have the prescription filled.

Anticonvulsant drugs such as Dilantin (for epilepsy) fluctuate greatly in the body, and it takes only a minute overdose to cause severe damage. Gentamicin (an antibiotic) can cause deafness unless it is monitored carefully. Anticoagulant drugs must also be monitored regularly (see **Prothrombin Time**), as must drugs used in arthritis (see **Salicylates**).

Toxicology involves not only testing for overdose of a drug (see **Barbiturates**; **Bromides**) but also monitoring for the optimal therapeutic effect (see **Digitalis Toxicity**). Antibiotic drugs, psychotherapeutic agents such as tranquilizers and antidepressants, and vitamins are also monitored regularly. In most instances blood is taken from a vein and the serum is tested. Urine, body tissues, and even hair or nail shavings are sometimes tested.

When performed: To assure that therapeutic blood levels are reached; to prevent toxic reactions from drugs *before* symptoms develop; to detect overdose or abuse of a drug; to determine why a patient does not respond to a drug.

Normal values: Normal values are those that produce a therapeutic effect without causing toxicity. When theophylline drugs (for asthma) are used, they must reach a certain level in the blood before they are effective; less than the required amount in the blood is the same as no drug at all.

Abnormal values: A detectable amount of drug greater than that needed to produce a therapeutic effect is considered abnormal. For example, when Dilantin is prescribed, the drug is given in dosages to produce a blood concentration of from 10 to 20 mcg per ml. Should the blood levels go above 20 mcg per ml, toxicity will occur. Although the therapeutically effective dose of a drug may vary with the size of an individual, the amount of a drug in the blood that can cause toxicity usually remains consistent.

DRUNK DRIVER, see *Alcohol*

DRY EYE, see *Schirmer's*

DSR, see *Radiography*

DWARFISM, see *Growth Hormone*

DYNAMIC EXERCISE CARDIOGRAM, see *Electrocardiogram*

DYNAMIC SPATIAL RECONSTRUCTOR, see *Radiography*

EAR BALANCE, see *Caloric*

ECG, see *Electrocardiogram*

ECHOCARDIOGRAM

The echocardiogram is considered by many physicians to be almost equal in value to the standard **Electrocardiogram** (ECG). Echocardiography is based on the principles of underwater detection (sonar) that the Navy developed during World War II. When a sound wave is directed into the heart at various locations, the echo, or rebounding sound wave, graphically reflects each part of the heart off which it bounces (see **Ultrasound**). Analysis of the echo images allows a three-dimensional "visualization" of the heart, the heart valves, the muscular structures, and even the blood as it passes through. The technique is similar to fluoroscopy, but with far more detail and with no radiation exposure (the sound waves used to obtain the echos have never been shown to be harmful).

A transducer (an instrument that can transmit energy into sound and also simultaneously receive sound and translate it back into energy that can be visualized) is rubbed over the heart area of the chest. (Usually a coating of mineral oil is applied to the chest to prevent air from seeping between the instrument and the body.) The transducer can be directed to any specific heart area, and the recorded echo patterns detail the opening and closing and condition of the heart valves. Echocardiograms can also indicate the size of each heart chamber, whether there are any masses in the heart, and especially whether there is excess fluid in the sac around the heart (pericardial effusion)—usually the result of infection or irritation from disease adjacent to the heart.

When performed: To diagnose heart valve disease, enlarged heart, heart tumors, and especially congenital heart defects in infants; when pericardial effusion is suspected; in instances of chest pain, fever, and fainting that cannot be diagnosed; to follow the progress of patients with heart valve replacements.

Normal values: Extensive experience is required to interpret echocardiograms, and great skill and knowledge of heart anatomy are needed to direct the sound waves properly. Thus normal values depend primarily on the technique of the test and the ability of the cardiologist to read the results. Multiple layers of thick and thin lines reflect the echoes from the various layers of heart structure that receive the sounds. There are specific measurements in centimeters (cm) for each area—such as the thickness of the heart wall or the heart chamber (when filled and when empty)—as well as normal expectations of how much blood the heart should hold and eject each time it beats. The difference between normal and abnormal may, however, be only a slight variation in the thickness of one sound wave lasting less than 0.1 second.

Abnormal values: A cardiologist can detect a defect in the opening and closing of a heart valve as well as structural defects in all areas of the heart. The picture of an abnormality can help indicate when certain kinds of treatment will be successful.

ECHOENCEPHALOGRAM, see *Ultrasound*

ECHOGRAM, see *Ultrasound*

EDROPHONIUM, see *Tensilon*

EEG, see *Electroencephalogram*

EJACULATE, see *Semen*

EKG, see *Electrocardiogram*

ELECTROCARDIOGRAM (ECG)

The electrocardiogram, or ECG (formerly known as the EKG because of the original German spelling of the word: **Electrokardiagramma**), is a graphic measure of the heart's muscular activity and a reflection of the self-generated electrical impulses that pass through the heart muscle, causing contraction and relaxation. Various electrodes called leads are placed on the body, usually one on each wrist and ankle and one on the chest that can be moved over the entire heart area. (The leads are metal contacts capable of detecting electrical activity within the body; they do not give off any electricity or have any activity of their own.)

By employing any two electrodes and greatly magnifying the activity they detect, the physician can obtain a diagrammatic representation of the heart's activity. If, for example, the lead from the right arm and the left leg are used, the ECG will largely reflect the activity of the right side of the heart; the same results will be obtained if the movable chest lead is placed to the right of the sternum (breastbone). Use of the various leads in different combinations offers many different "views" of the heart; 12 different "views" are considered standard or routine.

The recorded electrocardiograph shows the rate and regularity of the heart's rhythm; it can also show the force or effectiveness of each heartbeat; the extent and location of any heart muscle damage (both old and new), and the effect of certain drugs. Unfortunately, the ECG can also give false readings; that is, the graph may show what seem to be abnormalities when the heart is normal, or it may fail to reveal heart damage when present. It is not a perfect test and is usually accompanied by several other tests for confirmation of a diagnosis.

For example, when the ECG appears to be normal but the patient has complaints referable to the heart, a stress ECG (sometimes called a treadmill test, an exercise ECG, or a dynamic exercise ECG) may be performed. With the ECG leads in place, the patient walks on a treadmill at a set speed and incline (or operates a stationary bicycle); the ECG is recorded while exercising. Normally no change is observed other than an expected increase in the rate of the heart. But in some patients the extra physical activity cuts down the amount of oxygen reaching the heart muscle, and this shows up on the ECG. The test is stopped immediately if oxygen shortage occurs.

The oldest type of exercise test is the Master two-step (devised by Dr. Arthur Master), in which a patient walks up and down two steps for a specified number of times while the ECG is recorded. This is still an effective test, but it has been replaced by the more impressive treadmills. The stress ECG is considered by some physicians to be a fair predictor of future heart problems. But many physicians feel that the test has no value. Studies have shown that two out of three patients without symptoms who take an exercise ECG may have a false positive result; that is, heart disease may be indicated erroneously.

Another form of heart stress testing is the quiz electrocardiogram. While the ECG is being recorded, the patient is asked questions that both threaten his ego and provoke anxiety. Changes in the ECG during the questioning period can indicate emotionally caused heart disease.

A more recent innovation of the ECG is the Holter monitoring test, in which the patient wears a tiny, portable ECG recording machine (sometimes combined with a tiny voice tape recorder) for 24 hours and notes (or records) any unusual stresses during the day as well as all normal activities (eating, going to the bathroom, etc. This test can isolate previously hidden heart disease and, of even greater importance, can help indicate causative factors such as personality problems.

Another new method of testing heart function is the SHK-STI (Spodick-Haffty-Kotilainen measurement and calculation of the **Systolic Time Intervals**). The patient wears an earpiece containing a photoelectric cell that measures the velocity of the blood entering and leaving the ear at the same time that chest electrodes are recording the ECG. These measurements of how well the heart is functioning can be made over a 24-hour period and can be correlated with normal physical activity and exercise.

When performed: The test is performed whenever heart disease is suspected and often as a routine checkup. (It is advisable to have at least one ECG before the age of 40 in order to note any changes that may occur at a later date.) It is also performed whenever a patient complains of shortness of breath, intermittent chest pain, or "palpitations," and when patients are taking drugs such as digitalis or diuretics (which tend to cause potassium changes that can severely affect the heart's activity).

Normal values: Each lead of the ECG has a fairly normal but slightly different pattern. The rate of the heart should be between 70 and 100 beats per minute (athletes may have normal rates of 50), and the pattern should be regular (no extra or missed beats).

Abnormal values: Extensive training and experience in interpreting ECGs allow the physician to detect even a slight variation from normal or expected patterns. The changes may indicate a muscle defect (either damage or insufficient oxygen), or they may reveal nerve conduction changes, which can come from damage to the heart arteries that bring oxygen to the heart muscle or damage to the muscle itself (from the aging process or from old infections). Enlargement of the heart, congenital defects, and valve disease may also be indicated by the ECG.

Note: See also **Apexcardiogram**; **Ballistocardiogram**; **Circulation Time**; **Echocardiogram**; **Phonocardiogram**; **Pulse Analysis**; **Radarkymogram**; **Systolic Time Intervals**; **Vectorcardiogram**.

ELECTROENCEPHALOGRAM (EEG)

The electroencephalogram is a graphic recording of the minute electric current given off by brain cell activity. The current is amplified, translated into wavy lines (waves), and recorded on paper. The waves represent intermittent brain cell activity; the height of the waves as well as the distance between each peak depends on body activity (for example, blinking or opening and closing the eyes can create seemingly abnormal waves). The waves can also show hyperactive brain cell activity as seen with epilepsy and interference with brain cell activity as seen with tumors.

From 10 to 24 electrodes are applied to the scalp in specific positions to aid in locating any abnormal lesion that might be reflected on the electroencephalograph. The patient lies quietly with eyes closed and no body movement. At times the patient is told to breathe fast and deeply, as this seems to amplify EEG waves.

The waves of brain activity recorded on the electroencephalograph are classified by Greek letters (alpha, beta, etc.). The biofeedback machine is essentially an electroencephalograph constructed to detect only alpha waves.

When performed: Whenever any nervous system or brain disease is suspected; whenever there are brief episodes of unconsciousness or fainting; following head injury; whenever a patient has suffered a convulsion; when there are persistent episodes of narcolepsy (falling asleep in the midst of one's usual activities).

Normal values: Alpha waves (with a frequency of 8 to 15 cycles per second) and beta waves (with a frequency of 16 to 30 cycles per second) are normally found in all individuals. The strength of the wave (the distance above and below the base line) is also important in making a diagnosis.

Abnormal values: Theta waves (with a frequency of 4 to 8 cycles per second) may be found in some normal individuals, but they should not make up more than 10% of the overall recording. An excess of theta waves can indicate a brain tumor, brain damage following a head injury, epilepsy, or stroke.

Delta waves (with a frequency of less than 4 cycles per second) are indicative of a very serious condition (severe injury, brain abscess, brain tumor, or massive brain hemorrhage). Severe infection (encephalitis) can also cause delta waves.

Other wave patterns are specific for epilepsy; often the type of epilepsy can be determined by the electroencephalograph.

ELECTROLYTES, see *Bicarbonate*; *Chloride*; *Potassium*; *Sodium*

ELECTROMYOGRAPHY (EMG)

Electromyography is a diagnostic neurologic test to study the potential (electrically measured activity) of muscle at rest, the reaction of muscle to contraction, and the response of muscle to insertion of a needle. The test is an aid in ascertaining whether a patient's illness is directly affecting the spinal cord, muscles, or peripheral nerves.

The patient lies at rest while the peripheral nerves in various areas are stimulated through electrodes, and the electrical activity in muscles and nerves is recorded. In needle electromyography, a small needle is inserted into the muscle and the patient is observed for electrical activity in the muscle at rest, on insertion of the needle, and during muscle contraction. The test is sometimes employed as a measure of the muscle tension produced by nervous stress; usually the muscles of the forehead are tested, since they can indicate relaxation or generalized body tension.

When performed: To aid in the diagnosis of diseases affecting the muscles, peripheral nerves, and spinal cord; to detect "hysterical" weakness and paralysis.

Normal values: Normally when the muscle is at rest, no electrical activity is observed. When muscles contract, the electromyograph shows a smooth graphic wave-like representation of each contraction; the graph lines are amplified with the increase in strength of each contraction.

Abnormal values: Muscle disease produces a spiked wave pattern; the shape of the spike depends on the particular disease. Muscle weakness produces a diminished wave. With myasthenia gravis, the waves disappear after a few minutes. Nerve involvement as opposed to muscle involvement usually shows a decreased frequency of contractions.

ELSBERG, see *Smell Function*

EMG, see *Electromyography*

EMMETROPIA, see *Visual Acuity*

ENCEPHALITIS, see *Complement Fixation*

ENDOSCOPY

More than 100 years ago a doctor put an open tube into the esophagus of a patient and, using the light from an oil lamp, was able to inspect the esophagus walls. This was the first instance of endoscopy—direct observation of a body organ or cavity. Since that time, the simple, open tubes have been replaced by far more intricate "scopes"; the latest, called fiberoptic endoscopes, can bend light rays so that the doctor can see around corners and obstacles and pinpoint the exact location of any pathology.

The endoscope is now used to examine the esophagus, the stomach, and even the intestines. The instrument is usually equipped not only to allow for observation but also to pump air into the cavity so as to extend the walls and make observation easier; to wash away anything that may obstruct the view (such as blood when looking for a bleeding ulcer); to suction out suspected material for **Cytology** tests; and to take a **Biopsy** specimen for testing. For examination of the upper gastrointestinal tract, the patient usually swallows the tip of the instrument (after the throat has been sprayed with local anesthesia); the swallowed tip carries the narrow tubing along with it.

A similar type of instrument used to detect lung disease is called a bronchoscope; the bronchoscope is usually equipped with a whirling brush at the tip to pick up bronchial cells under a thick mucous layer for microscopic study. Use of the proctosigmoidoscope in the rectum and large bowel is yet another form of endoscopy. Newer colonoscopes can reach as far as five feet into the lower intestinal tract.

At times a direct incision is made in the skin and an endoscope is inserted to view the area beneath. When this is done in the portion of the chest just above the breastbone, it is called mediastinoscopy. This form of endoscopy enables the physician to view the bronchi from the outside, the large blood vessels as they enter and emerge from the heart, and the lymph nodes in the area (which are especially diagnostic when looking for certain tumors).

When the incision for an endoscope is made over the abdomen, it is called peritoneoscopy or laparoscopy. Direct examination of the abdominal cavity offers a unique way of testing the liver for size, growth, and clotting defects, and for obtaining a tissue specimen. With abdominal endoscopy it is also possible to see the gall bladder, pancreas, and spleen, along with the ovaries and outer surface of the uterus.

Hysteroscopy is an endoscopic test that allows direct examination of the inside of the uterus. Cystoscopy refers to direct examination of the inside of the bladder; vaginoscopy offers a more detailed scrutiny of the vagina than can be obtained by the usual techniques. Recently the endoscope has been adapted to look into joints; knee endoscopy allows a specific test to evaluate meniscus cartilage or ligament tears of that joint. (Doctors can now perform corrective surgery on the knee through the endoscope.) In almost all instances, endoscopy is performed in conjunction with X-rays (see **Radiography**).

When performed: When X-rays show suspected lesions in an area that can ultimately be viewed directly by an endoscope (such as bleeding stomach ulcer or liver abscess); when congenital malformations are suspected in various organs, especially the esophagus; when growths, abscesses, or inadequate functioning of an organ is suspected; whenever a biopsy is needed to confirm a diagnosis; when there is abdominal or chest pain that cannot be explained; following trauma when internal injuries are suspected.

Normal values: When an organ (or the surface or lining of an organ) is viewed directly, it should appear normal to the examining physician. Normal values are based primarily on extensive experience (only a trained eye can spot a pinpoint lesion or ulcer).

Abnormal values: Evidence of tumor, abscess, blocked or nonfunctioning ducts, infection, or hemorrhage is considered abnormal.

EOM, see *Strabismus*

EPILEPSY, see *Electroencephalogram*; *Manganese*

EPILEPSY DRUG, see *Drug Monitoring*

EPINEPHRINE, see *Catecholamines*

EPT, see *Pregnancy*

ER, see *Estrogen Receptor*

ERYTHROCYTE, see *Red Blood Cell*

ERYTHROCYTE HEMOLYSIS, see *Tocopherols*

ERYTHROCYTE INDICES, see *Red Blood Cell Indices*

ERYTHROCYTE SEDIMENTATION RATE, see *Sedimentation Rate*

ESOPHAGEAL X-RAY, see *Radiography*

ESOPHAGOSCOPY, see *Endoscopy*

ESR, see *Sedimentation Rate*

ESTROGEN (Estradiol, Estrone, Estriol)

Estrogens are really several different female hormones comprised of estradiol (the most potent), estrone, and estriol. All the estrogens are manufactured principally by the ovaries, but small amounts can come from the adrenal glands and even, in men, from the testicles. Usually the total amount of estrogens is measured in the urine; individual components may also be tested. Estradiol can be measured in blood plasma taken from a vein. Estrogen production is controlled by the pituitary gland and responds not only to pregnancy and phases of the menstrual cycle but also to stress (anxiety) situations.

When performed: When little or no ovary function is suspected; when pituitary gland dysfunction is suspected; during pregnancy; when certain inherited sexual dysfunctions are under consideration; when a woman has excessive menstruation that cannot easily be explained; in cases of infertility.

Normal values: Nonpregnant women usually secrete from 10 to 60 mcg of total estrogen per 24-hour urine sample during the first two weeks of the menstrual cycle; this amount rises to about 100 mcg per 24 hours of urine during the last two weeks of the cycle. In pregnant women 24-hour urinary estrogen may rise to 40,000 mcg. Children secrete less than 1 mcg per day. After menopause 1 to 20 mcg per day is normal. Men normally secrete up to 20 mcg in a 24-hour urine sample.

The normal range of plasma estradiol varies with phases of the menstrual cycle. During the first 10 days it averages 50 pg per ml; during the last 20 days it averages 125 pg per ml. Men normally average 20 pg per ml at all times.

Abnormal values: Elevated urinary estrogen levels can result from ovarian tumors, excessive pituitary activity (which can also come from hypothalamic pathology), adrenal hyperactivity, liver disease, and certain inherited chromosomal abnormalities. A decreased amount of estrogens can be found when a patient takes female hormones (which stop body manufacture of estrogens), with problems during pregnancy, with decreased pituitary activity, and with ovarian failure.

Usually, when abnormal values of estrogens are discovered, specific tests for the various components of estrogen are performed to ascertain the cause. (When a patient takes diethylstilbestrol, for example, the estriol portion of estrogen decreases.) Recently estrogen measurements have also been taken in men; an elevated level (especially of plasma estradiol) with reduced testosterone (see **Testis Function**) seems to be a risk factor in heart disease.

ESTROGEN RECEPTOR (ER)

Some cancers of the breast, uterus, ovary, skin, lymph nodes, and stomach "respond" to and can be treated by certain hormones. It is of great advantage to know which cancers will react to hormone therapy. Two out of three cancer tissues that will absorb estrogens (and an even higher ratio of tissues that also absorb progesterones—progesterone receptor) can be treated by various forms of hormonal manipulation and antiestrogen drugs in place of surgery. The Estrogen Receptor test measures the response of a tumor to estrogen stimulation.

In the estrogen receptor test, a tiny specimen of body tissue (see **Biopsy**), usually breast, is studied to see how responsive it is to estrogens—how it reacts (grows or diminishes) to the hormone's activity in the body. This test is a particular measure of whether a tumor is hormone-sensitive and thus whether it would be of value to have the patient's adrenals or pituitary gland removed (or destroyed by radiation) as part of therapy.

When performed: To ascertain if a cancer can be treated with hormones; when a patient has a metastatic (spreading throughout the body) cancer whose source cannot be located but the cancer itself can be biopsied to indicate if it is treatable by drugs; to show which cancer patients will not benefit from certain surgical procedures such as removal of the pituitary gland or adrenal glands; to indicate which cancer patients might benefit from chemotherapy.

Normal values: There are no normal values for this test; when more than 3 femtomoles of the protein estrogen receptor are found in a cancer, it is considered positive or hormone-receptive.

Abnormal values: A negative response, or failure of the tissue to indicate the presence of estrogen receptors, usually means that hormone treatment will not work and that chemotherapy should be tried.

ETHANOL, see *Alcohol*

ETHYL ALCOHOL, see *Alcohol*

ETHYLENE GLYCOL, see *Methanol*

EXCLUSION OF PARENTHOOD, see *Disputed Parentage*

EXERCISE CARDIOGRAM, see *Electrocardiogram*

EXOPHTHALMOMETER

The exophthalmometer measures the exact amount of eyeball protrusion, called exophthalmos. Most often "bulging" eyeballs (an excess of the white part of the eye showing) occur in patients with hyperthyroidism. But other diseases can also cause either one or both eyes to protrude. The exophthalmometer (an instrument similar to the device used to measure pupil distance when fitting eyeglasses) is placed in front of the eyes, and the amount of protrusion is measured for each eye.

When performed: When thyroid disease is suspected; when sinus disease, cancer, brain disease, eye infection, or various blood and blood vessel diseases are suspected; when glaucoma is suspected but not found.

Normal values: Eyeball protrusion should not exceed 15 mm.

Abnormal values: Protrusion greater than 16 mm is considered abnormal, especially when one eye protrudes more than the other. Once thyroid disease is eliminated from the diagnosis, special examinations such as X-rays (see **Radiography**), blood tests, and tests for infection are employed. Patients with severe nearsightedness or retraction of the eyelids (either naturally or as a consequence of cosmetic surgery) may appear to have protruding eyes, but this is not an indication of disease.

EXTERNAL OCULAR MUSCLE, see *Strabismus*

EYE, see *Visual Acuity*

EYE SONOGRAM, see *Ultrasound*

FACIAL RECOGNITION

Testing for the ability to differentiate between pictures of unfamiliar faces (and to remember the characteristics of such faces) has been found to be a fairly reliable way to distinguish organic (physical) brain disease from problems of a psychological nature. Patients with real brain pathology cannot discriminate between different unfamiliar faces and have great difficulty remembering an unfamiliar face they have seen several minutes earlier. Patients who pretend to have certain diseases and those with neurotic problems tend to remember faces in such a test and can repeatedly tell one from another. Patients are shown frontal and profile views of unfamiliar faces (photographed under varying light conditions) and are asked to remember them so as to identify other pictures that are of the same person.

When performed: To help differentiate between neurological and psychological conditions, especially when brain disease is suspected.

Normal values: Normal test scores range from 36 to 54 (a perfect score).

Abnormal values: A definite abnormal score is 35 or less and usually indicates physical brain damage. Patients with schizophrenia usually have normal scores.

FARSIGHTEDNESS, see *Visual Acuity*

FASTING BLOOD SUGAR, see *Glucose*

FECES EXAMINATION

The average adult excretes approximately 100 to 300 g (3 to 10 ounces) of fecal matter per day, of which about 70% may be water. The feces (stool) can offer valuable diagnostic clues to diseases of the bowel, the blood, and the metabolic system, and especially to infectious processes that cannot be diagnosed.

Many tests can be performed on the feces. The usual examination consists of noting the color and the presence or absence of blood and mucus, and then making a microscopic search for parasites (worms, amoeba) and their eggs (ova) and a culture for bacteria. On occasion, the amount of fat is measured after a patient is given a high-fat diet for three days. Patients should not brush their teeth or eat meat for three days prior to the test, since any traces of blood from the gums or from rare meat in the feces can cause a false positive reaction.

The Scotch tape test is used to find worms that come out of the bowel at night (particularly pinworms). A piece of Scotch tape is wrapped around a pencil, sticky side out, and touched to the anal area after the body has been warmed, usually under a blanket. The tape is then placed on a glass slide and examined under the microscope.

When performed: As a routine or screening test to detect unsuspected (very early stage) gastrointestinal disease; in an undiagnosed infection (diarrhea); when there is an undiagnosed metabolic difficulty (weight loss); as a verification of gall bladder disease.

Normal values: The normal color of feces (although a great deal depends on diet) ranges from light to dark brown. Microscopic examination should show a predominance of partly digested foods and only a rare blood cell or shred of mucus. Less than 25% of the feces' dry weight should be fat. No parasites or their eggs should be present.

Abnormal values: When there is gall bladder or liver disease, the feces acquires a gray to gray-white color. If there is bleeding high up in the bowel (from the esophagus to the small intestine), the feces have a black, tarry appearance; if the bleeding is near the rectum, red blood may be seen. Yellow-colored feces are seen with certain digestive diseases, especially of the pancreas (sprue). Following a bout of food poisoning, the feces may acquire a greenish hue. Beets can color the stool red.

Any amount of blood (even occult: not visible but measurable) in the feces is abnormal. Its presence indicates bleeding somewhere in the gastrointestinal system and can mean cancer, infection, anemia, or injury to the bowel.

It is abnormal for more than 25% of the solid part of the stool sample to be fat. Increased amounts of fat in the feces are seen with pancreatic disease, biliary tract obstruction, and problems of intestinal absorption.

An increased amount of mucus is seen in many gastrointestinal conditions, especially infection, dysentery, colitis, fistula, and pancreatic disease.

Microscopic examination of the stool sample can show a specific parasite or its egg that may be causing unknown fever, weight loss, and unusual fatigue. Worm infestation can cause asthmatic symptoms.

FEMALE HORMONE, see *Estrogen*

FEMALE-MALE IDENTITY, see *Chromatin*

FEMINIZING, see *Cortisol*

FERRIC CHLORIDE, see *Phenylketonuria*

FERRITIN, see *Iron*

FETAL HEMOGLOBIN, see *Hemoglobin*

FEVER BLISTER, see *Herpes*

FIBRINOGEN

Fibrinogen (Factor I), a plasma protein manufactured in the liver, is one of the 12 known primary factors essential to the clotting of blood. After a patient suffers an injury that causes bleeding, thromboplastin is given off by damaged tissues and combines with prothrombin and calcium in the body to form thrombin. The thrombin then combines with fibrinogen to make the fibrous substance that allows clot formation. Inability to form fibrinogen may be inherited or acquired from disease. Blood is taken from a vein and the plasma is tested.

When performed: When a coagulation defect (inability of the blood to clot) is suspected; with excessive unexplained black-and-blue areas or mucous membrane bleeding.

Normal values: Normal fibrinogen levels range from 200 to 500 mg per 100 ml or 0.2 to 0.5 g per 100 ml.

Abnormal values: Deficiency of fibrinogen (hypofibrinogenemia) may be congenital as well as acquired from liver disease, vitamin B deficiency, and certain bone cancers. Fibrinogen levels may be elevated in nephrosis and multiple myeloma. In pregnancy and in certain severe infections, the levels are slightly higher than normal.

FIELD OF VISION, see *Visual Field*

FINGER WRINKLE

The autonomic nervous system controls many functions of the body (heart rate, blood pressure, circulation, bronchial tube relaxation, sweating). One part of the system, the sympathetic nervous system, causes adrenalin and similar substances to be produced. The functioning of the sympathetic nerves is tested by placing the patient's hands in warm water for at least half an hour and noticing if the skin of the fingers wrinkles after the soaking.

When performed: When there is suspicion of Raynaud's disease (blockage of artery circulation, usually in the extremities), diabetes, or Guillain-Barré disease (pathology of the nerves).

Normal values: The skin of the fingers will normally wrinkle after being soaked in water.

Abnormal values: With diseases of the sympathetic nervous system, the skin does not wrinkle after soaking. After a sympathectomy (a surgical procedure

THE ENCYCLOPEDIA OF

to sever the sympathetic nerves, usually performed in patients with poor circulation), the skin will not wrinkle on the operated side.

FISHBERG, see *Mosenthal*

FLOCCULATION, see *Agglutination*

FLUORESCEIN EYE STAIN

Fluorescein, an orange-colored dye, is used in testing for abnormalities of the cornea (the surface over the pupil and lens of the eye). The dye is dropped onto the eye and allowed to spread over the surface. Sometimes individual sterile strips of paper containing the dye are used instead of liquid fluorescein to avoid the possibility of bacterial growth in the bottled solution. The dye will lodge in any irregularities on the cornea, the rest will wash away with tears. When ultraviolet or "black" light is then directed on the eye, the fluorescein will glow green and so indicate any abnormalities such as scratches, ulcers, foreign bodies (even as small as an eyelash hair), and various infectious diseases that can cause physical damage to the corneal surface.

Most eye injuries and other problems can be observed directly by the physician when the ultraviolet light is directed on the eye; in addition, a biomicroscope or "slit lamp" may be used to obtain a greatly magnified view of the eye surface. The biomicroscope is also used for more detailed examination of the structures of the eye.

When performed: Whenever any injury to or infection of the eye is suspected, especially when a superficial examination shows no evidence of trauma: during and after the fitting of contact lenses to make sure that tears pass normally under each lens; before applying cortisone to the eye.

Normal values: If there is no break in the surface of the cornea either from disease or injury, the fluorescein stain will wash out with tears and will reflect no damage when subjected to ultraviolet light.

Abnormal values: Any break in the smooth corneal surface will show a greenish fluorescence when viewed under ultraviolet light. From the size, shape, and location of the dye, the physician can usually make a specific diagnosis.

FLUORESCENT TREPONEMAL ANTIBODY, see *Syphilis*

FLUOROSCOPY, see *Radiography*

FOLATES (Folic Acid)

Folates, of which folic acid is but one version, are essential to prevent anemia. Large amounts are found in beef, green vegetables, liver, nuts, oranges, and yeast. They become reduced primarily from an inadequate diet, but also from alcoholism and certain drugs such as birth control pills. The body stores of folic acid last for only a month or two, and folate deficiency can often be diagnosed before anemia is apparent. Blood is drawn from a vein and the serum is examined.

When performed: When folic acid deficiency, especially in pregnancy, or megaloblastic anemia (abnormally large but undeveloped red blood cells) is suspected; when the tongue is smooth and enlarged.

Normal values: Normal folic acid levels range from 5 to 25 ng per ml of serum.

Abnormal values: Decreased folic acid levels in the serum are found in malnutrition, pregnancy, anemia, alcoholism, and intestinal diseases characterized by malabsorption of folic acid (such as celiac disease and sprue).

FOLIC ACID, see *Folates*

FOOD-COLORING ALLERGY, see *Tartrazine Sensitivity*

FORCED EXPIRATORY VOLUME, see *Pulmonary Function*

FORCED VITAL CAPACITY, see *Pulmonary Function*

FORSSMAN ANTIBODY, see *Mononucleosis*

FRANKLINIC, see *Taste Function*

FREE FATTY ACIDS, see *Lipids*

FREE THYROXINE, see *Thyroid Function*

FRIEDMAN, see *Pregnancy*

FTA-ABS, see *Syphilis*

FUNCTIONAL RESIDUAL CAPACITY, see *Pulmonary Function*

FUNDOSCOPY

The fundus, or back part of the eyeball, is examined by using an ophthalmoscope. The primary area examined is the retina (which receives images and transmits them to the brain); this is also the only area of the body where blood vessels (small arteries and veins) can be seen directly. The optic disc—the point where the optic nerve enters the brain from the eye—is also examined; the appearance of the edge or margin of this small, circular area is important in the diagnosis of many different diseases. Usually a tiny beam of light is projected through the pupil onto the back of the eyeball; the area is viewed through a variety of ophthalmoscopic lenses to focus upon the particular object being studied (blood vessel, retina, nerve).

When performed: Usually part of any routine physical examination by a physician as well as any eye exam by an ophthalmologist; when eye disease such as glaucoma is suspected; whenever diabetes, atherosclerosis (artery disease), or hypertension is suspected; when brain lesion or brain disease is considered; following head injury; to corroborate certain infections and malignancies.

Normal values: The optic disc, the retina, and the blood vessels should appear normal to the doctor. Specific terms are used to indicate the presence or absence of disease (such as stages of high blood pressure, diabetes, or the protrusion of the optic disc).

Abnormal values: Abnormal values depend on the degree of disease observed through the ophthalmoscope and are usually rated from I to V, depending on severity.

FUNGUS

Diseases caused by fungi (molds and yeasts) are called mycotic. They can cause localized problems such as the tiny, itching white patches that sometimes appear in the mouth, throat, or vagina; or they can be the basis for extremely serious, sometimes fatal systemic body infections such as coccidioidomycosis and cryptococcosis. Ringworm is a fungus disease; common forms include athlete's foot and, when in the groin, "jock itch."

The easiest way to test for a fungus is to take a scraping or smear from the affected area and examine the specimen under the microscope; each fungus has a characteristic appearance. All take on a blue color when studied with the **Gram Stain** test. Some of the ringworm fungi will fluoresce (give off a greenish or brownish glow) when examined with Wood's light (ultraviolet rays), especially those on the scalp or under the nails.

When systemic illness or a blood infection is suspected, the blood from a vein is cultured to isolate the causative organism; it can sometimes take weeks before definitive growth of the disease-causing organism is seen. In rare instances, specimens thought to contain fungi are injected into animals to observe the effects (fungi develop much faster in animals than in humans). A specimen from the animal can then be tested to determine the kind of fungus growth.

When performed: Most commonly on areas of itching skin, especially the scalp; with persistent vaginal discharge; with persistent lung infections; with undiagnosed generalized infections, especially meningitis.

Normal values: Normally fungi are not found in or on the human body. On occasion, a nondisease-causing fungus may be isolated from the mouth or vagina. Such infestations usually do not last very long.

Abnormal values: The isolation of any pathological fungi from the skin, hair, or blood or under the nails is considered abnormal. Fungus diseases may be confirmed by **Skin Reaction**, **Agglutination**, and **Complement Fixation** tests.

GALL BLADDER VISUALIZATION, see *Radiography*

GALLIUM SCAN, see *Nuclear Scanning*

GAMMA CAMERA, see *Nuclear Scanning*

GAMMA GLUTAMYL TRANSFERASE, see *Alcoholism*

GASTRIC ANALYSIS

Gastric analysis is performed primarily to determine whether the stomach secretes hydrochloric acid (as it normally should); the test also shows whether the stomach produces the necessary digestive enzymes and whether it contains any cancer cells. Water, electrolytes, hydrochloric acid, mucin, pepsin, **gastrin**, and a substance called intrinsic factor that is necessary to absorb vitamin B_{12} are all components of gastric secretions. When a patient is at rest, only small amounts of acid are secreted. The sight and smell of food, as well as actual food intake, can cause the stomach to secrete acid.

A tube is passed through the nose or mouth and into the stomach. The gastric fluid is withdrawn by suction continually for one hour. (The patient should not eat or take any medication for 12 hours prior to the test.) If at the end of one hour there is still doubt about whether acid is being secreted, an injection of histamine may be given to stimulate maximal acid production. One hour later, the gastric fluid is again tested. A tubeless method of analysis (which is not as exact but more comfortable for the patient) may be performed by having the patient swallow a dye (Diagnex blue) and noting the color of the urine.

The stomach fluid of newborn infants is sometimes examined within 6 hours after birth to help diagnose the respiratory distress syndrome (breathing difficulty). The presence of lung fluid in gastric contents is considered positive for the disease.

When performed: Whenever there is an undiagnosed anemia or repeated stomach infections (gastritis); when certain vitamin deficiencies are suspected; when searching for stomach cancer; when tuberculosis is suspected but the tuberculosis bacteria cannot be found.

After ulcer surgery, insulin is sometimes injected into a patient to see if stomach acid is still being secreted. Normally insulin causes acid to appear, and absence of acid is a measure of the success of the surgery, which should have prevented acid formation.

Normal values: The average gastric hydrochloric acid output is 1.25 to 4 mEq per hour, but it can go as high as 12 mEq per hour and still be normal. Normal gastric secretory volume (all components) is between 50 and 100 ml per hour.

Abnormal values: Acid secretion is elevated in duodenal ulcer and in Zollinger-Ellison syndrome (gastrin-secreting tumor). In gastric cancer and anemia, less than the normal amount of acid (or no acid) is secreted.

Note: Gastric analysis should not be confused with a stomach contents examination. A stomach contents exam is occasionally performed (after washing out the stomach) to ascertain a poison or drug. It is commonly performed on a deceased person to help determine the time of death.

GASTRIN

In addition to acid and enzymes, the stomach produces a hormone called gastrin. This hormone, first provoked by eating food, causes the stomach lining to secrete hydrochloric acid. Gastrin also causes the pancreas to produce insulin and enzymes and the liver to produce bile, all of which aid in digestion. Finally, gastrin increases stomach and intestinal muscle activity, helping to move food down the intestinal tract. There are several other stomach hormones, but gastrin is the only one regularly tested for at this time. Blood is taken from a vein and the serum is measured.

When performed: When there are severe, seemingly incurable ulcers of the stomach and intestine; in cases of suspected pernicious anemia.

Normal values: Normal values range from 0 to 300 pg per ml; the amount seems to increase naturally as a person gets older and may reach 700 pg per ml.

Abnormal values: With the occasional exception of the elderly, any test value over 500 pg per ml is considered a sign of disease. When a stomach ulcer is responding to treatment, gastrin levels will be normal; but in patients with Zollinger-Ellison syndrome (tumors that secrete gastrin and cause multiple ulcers) gastrin levels may rise to 300,000 pg per ml. To affirm the diagnosis, a trace of very dilute hydrochloric acid is given. With Zollinger-Ellison syndrome, the gastrin level stays the same; with anemia, it decreases markedly after the acid reaches the stomach.

GASTROINTESTINAL ENDOSCOPY, see *Endoscopy*

GASTROINTESTINAL SERIES, see *Radiography*

GDH, see *Alcoholism*

GENETIC SEX IDENTITY, see *Chromatin*

GERMAN MEASLES, see *Agglutination*

GESELL DEVELOPMENTAL SCHEDULE, see *Motor Development*

GGTP, see *Alcoholism*

GIEMSA, see *Malaria*

GIGANTISM, see *Growth Hormone*

GI SERIES, see *Radiography*

GLAUCOMA, see *Tonometry*

GLOBULIN, see *Albumin/Globulin*

GLOMERULAR FILTRATION RATE, see *Creatinine*

GLUCAGON

Glucagon, a hormone produced by the pancreas (which also produces insulin), converts protein and fat molecules into blood sugars to be used as energy. Glucagon also causes insulin to be released into the body. Blood is taken from a vein and the plasma is tested. Glucagon is sometimes injected into a patient to help diagnose excess glycogen (stored glucose). Glucose is the body's chief energy substance; it is stored primarily in the liver but also in muscles. Normally, after a patient receives glucagon, blood glucose will increase markedly.

When performed: When hypoglycemia (low blood sugar) is suspected; to assess the control of diabetes (whether a patient is well regulated); to aid in the diagnosis of a type of pancreatic tumor that occurs primarily in women after the menopause and that causes a distinctive skin rash and weakness.

Normal values: Glucagon levels in plasma range from 60 to 100 pg per ml.

Abnormal values: Glucagon values are greatly increased with tumor of the pancreas, uncontrolled diabetes, and inadequate amounts of insulin. On occasion, glucagon is decreased with certain forms of hypoglycemia. It is also decreased after eating a large amount of carbohydrates.

GLUCOSE (Sugar)

The glucose test measures the amount of glucose floating free in the blood or excreted by the kidneys into the bladder. The test is really a measure of how well the body handles carbohydrate metabolism (the breakdown of starches such as vegetables as well as all the various sugar products in the foods we eat). Glucose is the primary fuel or energy source for all the body tissues. It may be burned directly or converted into fat and stored for later use as fatty acid energy. Glucose is stored primarily in the liver and, in small amounts, in other tissues. A uniform blood glucose level is generally maintained in the body through insulin secretion (which decreases it), despite variations due to dietary increase in sugar and energy expenditure. Blood is taken from the vein to assess the level of glucose in serum; glucose may also be tested in whole blood or plasma, in urine, or in spinal fluid.

In preparing for the glucose tolerance test (GTT), the patient eats his usual amount of carbohydrate for several days. Then he fasts for 8 to 12 hours prior to the test. First, a fasting blood glucose and urine glucose are measured. Then the patient is given 100 g of glucose in water or soda to drink. Thirty minutes afterward both the blood and urine are again examined for sugar levels. Glucose testing after eating is called postprandial. Every hour thereafter for the next five hours, urine and blood samples are taken to determine how long it takes the body to metabolize the 100 g of glucose. Sometimes the spinal fluid and joint fluids are tested for glucose. (Before more sophisticated methods of medical laboratory testing were developed, doctors used to taste their patient's urine for sugar.)

When performed: The fasting blood glucose is performed when there is dizziness, weakness, excessive thirst, excessive urination, or any other symptoms and signs suggesting diabetes. The test also helps diagnose hormone disorders, pancreatic disease, certain brain and spinal cord diseases, and many hereditary conditions. A single postprandial test may be performed as a confirmatory measure.

The glucose tolerance test is performed when the fasting and/or postprandial glucose determinations are borderline and diabetes or other disease is still being considered.

The urine examination for sugar is a routine screening test for diabetes as well as for suspected kidney, liver, or hormone disease.

Normal values: Fasting blood glucose levels normally range from 80 to 120 mg per 100 ml of serum, 60 to 100 mg per 100 ml of whole blood. Postprandial levels should not exceed 180 mg per 100 ml.

During the entire five to six hours of the glucose tolerance test, the peak should remain below 180 mg per 100 ml, and after two hours the levels should return to the same as for fasting.

In the urine sugar test, normally no sugar or only an insignificant trace should be detected, even after a high-carbohydrate meal. However, in some individuals who have a low kidney threshold, sugar may be detected in the urine without the presence of disease.

Abnormal values: The fasting blood glucose level is increased (hyperglycemia) with diabetes, Cushing's syndrome (pituitary disease), many endocrine problems, liver disease, and diuretic therapy. The level is decreased with pancreatic disorders, excessive insulin, and glycogen storage disease.

In order to justify a diagnosis of hypoglycemia as a disease condition, blood glucose levels must be less than 40 mg per 100 ml of serum in at least three different instances at the identical time the patient is having symptoms (sweating, palpitations, weakness, bizarre behavior). Alcohol intake may cause temporary hypoglycemia, as will fasting, liver disease, and certain cancers.

In the glucose tolerance test, levels are elevated for more than two hours with diabetes mellitus and decreased with pancreatitis, excess insulin production, and hypoglycemia.

Elevated levels of glucose in the urine may be caused by diabetes mellitus, liver disease, hyperthyroidism and other hormone disorders, pregnancy, brain injury, and excessive ingestion of sugar. In meningitis spinal fluid glucose is decreased; with joint infections joint fluid sugar is decreased.

GLUCOSE 6-PHOSPHATE DEHYDROGENASE (G6PD)

Glucose 6-phosphate dehydrogenase is an enzyme normally found in red blood cells. In people with a deficiency of this enzyme (an inherited condition), red blood cells are no longer protected from oxidation, causing hemolysis (destruction of red blood cells and subsequent separation of hemoglobin), which can lead to anemia. The deficiency is more frequent in Blacks, Orientals, and Caucasians from the Mediterranean area, and more serious in men than in women. Blood is taken from a vein and tested. It may simply be screened for the presence of G6PD, or the quantity of G6PD may be measured precisely. Either test can still miss the deficiency in some women.

When performed: In undiagnosed hemolytic anemia; before administration of antimalarial drugs, sulfonamides, and nitrofurans.

Normal values: Glucose 6-phosphate dehydrogenase should normally be found in significant amounts in red blood cells: 120 to 280 units per billion cells.

Abnormal values: Glucose 6-phosphate dehydrogenase deficiency, while not usually serious or chronic, can at times be fatal. It does not show itself until the patient ingests drugs or foods that precipitate the hemolytic anemia, which can then cause hemoglobinuria, jaundice, fever, and renal failure. Some of those drugs are Primaquine (for malaria), aspirin, sulfa products, nitrofurans, vitamin C, certain antibiotics, some worm medicines, inhalation of naphthalene (moth repellent), and eating fava beans—but only in people born with a G6PD deficiency.

GLUTAMATE DEHYDROGENASE, see *Alcoholism*

GLUTAMIC OXALACETIC TRANSAMINASE (SGOT)

Serum glutamic oxalacetic transaminase (SGOT) and serum glutamic pyruvic transaminase (SGPT) are enzymes present primarily in the heart and liver. (There are tiny amounts in the kidney, lungs, brain, and a few other body tissues.) These enzymes are unique in that they are released into the blood when there is heart muscle damage, liver cell destruction, or rickettsial (extra-large-size bacteria) infections. Blood is taken from a vein and the serum is tested.

When performed: When there is suspected heart damage; to follow the progress of a patient after a heart attack; in certain types of liver disease; when there is an unexplained infection.

Normal values: Normally there are less than 30 SGOT units per ml and less than 25 SGPT units per ml in the blood serum.

Abnormal values: Serum levels of SGOT and SGPT are elevated following a heart attack and reach their peak in 24 to 48 hours after the onset of illness. With heart disease, SGOT levels are higher than SGPT levels. Serum levels return to normal four to six days after the attack. In some acute heart disease (other than heart attack), the peak levels are reached in 72 hours. In liver disease (infectious hepatitis and cirrhosis) SGPT levels are higher than SGOT levels. Because a few other conditions such as pancreatitis, infectious mononucleosis, and certain muscle diseases can also cause an increase of these enzymes in the blood, they must always be evaluated along with the patient's symptoms.

Note: The newer name for SGOT is aspartate amino transferase (AST); SGPT is now called alanine amino transferase (ALT).

GLUTAMIC PYRUVIC TRANSAMINASE, see *Glutamic Oxalacetic Transaminase*

GLYCOHEMOGLOBIN

The glycohemoglobin test measures the percentage of hemoglobin molecules that have glucose (sugar) attached to them. The greater the amount of glucose in the blood, the greater the percentage of glycosylated hemoglobin (also known as Hb A1a-c). The test is of particular value in monitoring a patient with diabetes to ascertain that the patient's blood sugar level is properly controlled; thus it is also a measure of the success or failure of treatment.

Initially the glycohemoglobin test is usually performed along with the **Glucose** tolerance test; but it may be substituted for that test after a treatment regimen has been established, since it requires far less time and far fewer blood samples from the patient and since the patient need not fast beforehand. Glycohemoglobin measurements indicate blood sugar activity during the six to eight weeks prior to the test, whereas the glucose tolerance test measures only blood sugar levels at the moment. At the present time, the glycohemoglobin test is usually performed every two months in order to provide the physician with data to help control the diabetic patient. Blood from a vein is examined.

When performed: The test is used primarily to measure the control (proper treatment) of a patient with diabetes; it not only helps reveal difficulties in sugar utilization, but can also reveal patients who ignore their prescribed treatment. Sometimes the test is used to measure the body's carbohydrate metabolism.

Normal values: Patients without diabetes, and patients with the disease who are responding to treatment average from 2% to 7.5% glycohemoglobin.

Abnormal values: Patients who have uncontrolled diabetes or who are receiving inadequate treatment will have glycohemoglobin values greater than 7.5%. Values in excess of 9.2% indicate definite improper control of a diabetic condition. Rarely a patient with a known hemoglobin disease, but without diabetes, will have elevated values.

GLYCOSIDES, see *Digitalis Toxicity*

GLYCOSYLATED HEMOGLOBIN, see *Glycohemoglobin*

GONADOTROPIN, see *Pregnancy*; *Testis Function*

GOUT, see *Uric Acid*

GRAM STAIN

The Gram stain test (named after Dr. Hans Christian Gram, a Danish physician) is used primarily to distinguish various bacteria under the microscope that would otherwise be impossible to identify. Sputum, joint fluid, spinal fluid, urine, sinus discharge, urethral discharge, vaginal fluid, and exudates (ooze) from infections can all be examined in this manner. When the specimen takes a gentian violet (bluish purple) or safranin (red) stain, the morphology (size, shape, and form) of bacteria is more easily visualized and aids in both diagnosis and treatment. (Certain bacteria such as tuberculosis germs will not show up on the Gram stain and need special dyes.)

When performed: The test is used primarily to evaluate and distinguish infectious organisms in various body fluids and to aid in the precise choice of therapy. Certain antibiotics are effective only against Gram-positive organisms; other antibiotics are effective only against Gram-negative organisms.

Normal values: Normally no pathological bacteria are observed after staining.

Abnormal values: Gram-negative organisms stain an orange-red color and are usually representative of coliform-type (intestinal and urinary tract) diseases. Gram-positive organisms stain a bluish purple and are usually representative of streptococcal and staphylococcal (upper respiratory tract and abscess) diseases.

GRAVINDEX, see *Pregnancy*

GROWTH HORMONE

A pituitary gland hormone called somatotropin or human growth hormone (HGH) controls the height an individual attains. It is, of course, essential for normal growth. Testing for growth hormone offers the earliest indication of generalized pituitary problems. Blood is taken from a vein and the serum is tested. Several tests must be taken at different times before true values can be determined. At times it is necessary to give the patient a large amount of insulin (to produce hypoglycemia, or low blood sugar) to obtain accurate results. Today drugs are available to stop excessive growth hormone secretion (preventing gigantism, or abnormally tall individuals) as well as drugs to allow normal growth hormone secretion (preventing dwarfism).

When performed: The test is used whenever gigantism (acromegaly) or dwarfism is suspected. The earlier the test is performed and the abnormality revealed, the easier and more effective the treatment. The test is given, too, when hyperactive children take stimulant drugs such as dextroamphetamine or methylphenidate (Ritalin); these drugs seem to retard growth.

Normal values: Newborn infants usually have higher levels of somatotropin than adults (over 30 ng per ml); children generally average from 1 to 15 ng per ml; women average up to 30 ng per ml; and men usually range below 10 ng per ml. It is normal for growth hormone levels to increase after insulin is given and to decrease to near zero after a large amount of glucose (sugar) is consumed.

Abnormal values: Lower than normal values are found with dwarfism; elevated values appear with gigantism. Values may also be elevated with diabetes, in stressful situations, following surgery, and with infections. Taking female hormones will cause a rise in growth hormone levels.

G6PD, see *Glucose 6-Phosphate Dehydrogenase*

GUAIAC, see *Occult Blood*

GUTHRIE BACTERIAL INHIBITION ASSAY (GBIA), see *Phenylketonuria*

HAA, see *Australian Antigen*

HAM

HAM is a test for paroxysmal nocturnal hemoglobinuria, a disease that occurs in certain people after middle age. Symptoms include attacks of anemia, generalized aches and pains, chills, fever, and excessive amounts of hemoglobin in the urine as a consequence of hemolysis (destruction of defective red blood cells)—usually brought on during sleep. The specific cause of the condition is unknown, but it is believed to be a **Complement** reaction. Blood is taken from a vein and the serum is tested in an acid solution. A somewhat similar but less definitive test is the sugar water test (sucrose hemolysis test), in which the defective red cell, if present, dissolves in the presence of sucrose.

When performed: When paroxysmal nocturnal hemoglobinuria is suspected (usually because of an excess of hemoglobin in the urine on awakening); when a patient has repeated, severe infections that cannot be diagnosed; when there are undiagnosable pains, especially in the lower back or legs.

Normal values: Normally red blood cells do not hemolyze (dissolve and release their supply of hemoglobin) when mixed with a very mild acid solution or when exposed to a sugar (sucrose) solution.

Abnormal values: In patients with paroxysmal nocturnal hemoglobinuria, red blood cells break down when exposed to an acid solution with a **pH** of 6.7 or less or when placed in a sucrose solution.

HAPTOGLOBIN

Haptoglobin, a plasma globulin (see **Albumin/Globulin**), is a direct measure of

THE ENCYCLOPEDIA OF

hemolysis in the body. Hemolysis means a markedly increased breakdown of red blood cells and the liberation of **Hemoglobin** into the plasma; it can come about from disease, from certain inherited conditions, from certain drugs, and after snakebite. When hemolysis occurs, the red blood cells do not last as long as they should, and this usually (but not always) results in anemia. Blood is taken from a vein and the serum is tested.

When performed: When anemia is present, especially when it is thought to be from an inherited condition such as thalassemia (Mediterranean or Cooley's anemia) or from Rh problems; when it is suspected that certain environmental factors (chemicals, drugs, or physical injury) are causing anemia; in severe infections; with liver disease.

Normal values: Normal haptoglobin levels range from 50 to 150 mg per 100 ml of serum.

Abnormal values: As red blood cells are destroyed, the hemoglobin that is released combines with haptoglobin; thus reduced levels of haptoglobin indicate hemolysis, no matter what the specific cause. Decreased values of haptoglobin are also found in liver disease and with infectious mononucleosis. Certain severe infections, tissue damage such as with heart attack, and cancers cause increased haptoglobin levels.

HARDY-RAND-RITTLER, see *Color Blindness*

HARTNUP'S DISEASE, see *Aminoaciduria*

HB, see *Australian Antigen*

HbAla-c, see *Glycohemoglobin*

HBD, see *Hydroxybutyric Dehydrogenase*

HBsAg, see *Australian Antigen*

HCG, see *Pregnancy*; *Testis Function*

HCO3, see *Bicarbonate*

HCS, see *Placental Lactogen*

HDL, see *Cholesterol*; *Lipoproteins*

HEARING FUNCTION

Sound is heard in two different ways: by its intensity or volume (loudness) and by its tone, which depends on how fast or how slowly it vibrates. In tests of hearing ability, both factors are measured. In addition, patients are tested for the ability to hear sound by two different means of conduction: air conduction (sounds heard through the ear canal) and bone conduction (sounds detected by the bones around and behind the ear).

The simplest measures of hearing ability are the whisper and voice tests, in which the doctor, sitting about 20 feet away from the patient, whispers and then says numbers out loud while the patient listens with one ear covered. In the ticking-watch test, the physician notes how far away from the ear the watch is still heard.

The most precise hearing test is measured by the audiometer, a machine that puts out sounds of various tones and intensities (volumes). Pure tones vary from 64 cycles per second, or cps (very low, bass-type tones) to almost 12,000 cps (extremely shrill or high-pitched tones). The human ear can usually detect sounds from 16 to 16,000 cps (although some people can hear up to 20,000 cps). Many animals can hear tones of 50,000 cps, beyond the range of human hearing.

The intensity (volume) of sound is expressed in decibels (db). A whisper measures about 20 db. Background noise in the average home runs about 50 db; in an office, about 60 db. Loud classical music rates 80 db, rock music is more than 120 db, and a jet engine ranges from 140 to 180 db. Usually sounds greater than 130 db will cause pain.

For the air conduction part of the test, the patient wears earphones from the audiometer and listens to sounds of designated tones and intensities or to spoken words (sounds may also be broadcast through a speaker in a soundproof room). An attachment from the earphones is then applied to the bone behind the ear and hearing is tested via bone conduction. How well the patient hears sounds through air conduction is an indication of ear drum and middle ear function as well as ear-nerve disease. Bone conduction ability tests the function of the inner ear. **Tuning fork** tests may also be used to survey hearing problems and to confirm bone or nerve deafness.

When performed: Whenever there is difficulty in hearing, usually due to ear infection, an inherited condition, or excessive exposure to loud noises (as in certain occupations); following head injury.

Audiometer tests are now being performed in schools to screen out children with hearing loss at an early age.

Normal values: For screening purposes only, two pure tones of 256 cps and 4,096 cps (encompassing the range of normal speech sounds) at 5 to 10 db are transmitted through the earphones (air conduction). Should the patient have difficulty in hearing either of these sounds, a more detailed audiogram is performed. Normally, an individual can hear lower tones (64 cps) at 1 to 2 db, higher tones (11,584 cps) at about 10 db, and all pure tones in between at 10 db or less. Air conduction hearing is usually better than bone conduction hearing.

Abnormal values: The inability to hear pure tones below 10 db indicates inner-ear or nerve damage. There are many different kinds of deafness; some people lose only the ability to perceive high tones or low tones; some lose only air or bone conduction hearing. Following injury or excessive noise exposure, high-tone hearing is usually lost. When deafness is inherited, hearing for the entire range of tones is missing. Following infection, the speech range is most commonly lost. Certain antibiotic drugs cause nerve deafness; if the drugs are not used over too long a period of time, hearing may return, but in some instances the medication can cause permanent deafness.

Note: The Lombard test helps to detect faked hearing loss. While wearing audiometer earphones, a patient reads from a book; after a minute or two, a noise from the audiometer is sent to each ear. If hearing is normal, the reader's voice will become louder. Patients with true hearing loss will not raise their voices while reading.

HEART-DISEASE-PRONE PERSONALITY, see *Jenkins Activity Survey*

HEART SCAN, see *Nuclear Scanning*

HEMATOCRIT

The hematocrit shows the percentage of blood cells (mostly red blood cells) comprising the total blood volume. A blood sample from a vein is centrifuged (the solid matter is forced to the bottom of a specially marked tube, leaving the clear plasma in the upper section). In a sense, the test measures the viscosity (thickness) of the blood as well as the amount of fluid in the blood. Many doctors feel the hematocrit test is a better measure of anemia than the **Hemoglobin** test, especially if the patient's diet includes normal amounts of iron.

When performed: In diagnostic screening for anemias and dehydration; to follow the course of therapy for anemias and hemorrhage.

Normal values: Normal hematocrit readings range from 40% to 55% (slightly lower in women).

Abnormal values: Low hematocrit readings (decreased percentage of total cells) are found in red blood cell anemias, immediately after hemorrhage, and whenever there is excessive fluid intake. High hematocrit readings are found in severe dehydration and polycythemia, angina, and after surgery, trauma, or burns.

HEMIANOPIA, see *Visual Field*

HEMOCCULT, see *Occult Blood*

HEMOGLOBIN

There are many different forms of hemoglobin in the blood; these forms are usually measured together as the total hemoglobin. Hemoglobin is an iron protein substance manufactured inside newly forming red blood cells and stored there for the life of the cells. Because of its unique affinity for oxygen, its task is to pick up oxygen as the red blood cells pass through the lungs and deliver that oxygen to tissue cells throughout the body.

The amount of oxygen the blood can carry depends not only on the amount of hemoglobin present but also on its effectiveness. Exposure to toxic substances can alter the hemoglobin molecule; carbon monoxide gas will easily replace oxygen attached to hemoglobin and form carboxyhemoglobin, preventing any vital oxygen from reaching tissue cells. Carboxyhemoglobin turns the blood (and sometimes the skin) a brilliant red. The Katyama test distinguishes between carboxyhemoglobin and hemoglobin.

Methemoglobin forms when the red blood cells are exposed to certain drugs (especially non-prescription ones such as phenacetin and other aspirin substitutes) or to large amounts of nitrates that are used to treat heart disease and as food preservatives. Methemoglobin picks up oxygen but will not release it to the tissues, making the skin appear bluish. Aspirin-substitute drugs and certain laxatives containing sulfur can cause sulfhemoglobin; this differs from methemoglobin only in that it cannot be treated and stays in the blood until the red blood cells break down. Fetal hemoglobin is the oxygen-carrying iron in the fetus; it almost disappears in adulthood but remains in large quantities when there are various blood diseases. Hemoglobin S is associated with sickle cell disease. Iron in the diet is the primary source of hemoglobin; replacement iron is necessary when there is blood loss such as with injury or menstruation.

Whenever there is a decreased amount of hemoglobin in the body (the blood carries less oxygen), the heart usually compensates by increasing its effort to circulate blood (the pulse rate becomes more rapid). Only one drop of whole blood, which can be taken from the fingertip, earlobe, or heel, is needed for the test. Hemoglobin can, of course, be evaluated from blood taken for any other procedure. It is also looked for in urine as an indication of bleeding or poisoning.

When performed: Primarily when there is suspicion of anemia, no matter what kind or what the cause; to aid in the diagnosis of many inherited conditions; to distinguish certain poisonings from disease; as an indication of how much blood has been lost after injury or surgery.

Normal values: Total hemoglobin levels for men range from 14 to 18 g per 100 ml; for women, 12 to 15 g per 100 ml. Up to 1% carboxyhemoglobin or fetal hemoglobin may be present, but no more than 0.1% of methemoglobin or sulfhemoglobin should be detected. The urine should contain no hemoglobin.

Abnormal values: Serum hemoglobin is sometimes increased when red blood cells are suddenly damaged or destroyed, as with sickle cell disease or the Rh anemia of infancy. Polycythemia (a disease characterized by excessive red blood cells) may show increased hemoglobin.

Hemoglobin values are decreased in almost all forms of anemia, especially those associated with iron deficiency. Symptoms of anemia usually do not appear until the hemoglobin level goes below 8 g per 100 ml. Hemoglobin is decreased in leukemia, after hemorrhage, and in pregnancy (especially after delivery, when there is loss of blood).

Heavy cigarette smoking may cause carboxyhemoglobin values up to 20%, markedly reducing the amount of normal hemoglobin. Thus the test is often used as a check on people who smoke but who deny the fact.

HEMOGRAM, see *Blood Cell Differential*; *Hematocrit*; *Hemoglobin*; *Red Blood Cell*; *Red Blood Cell Indices*; *White Blood Cell*

HEMOLYSIS, see *Haptoglobin*

HEMOPHILIA, see *Partial Thromboplastin Time*

HEPARIN, see *Coagulometer*; *Partial Thromboplastin Time*

HEPATITIS-ASSOCIATED ANTIGEN, see *Australian Antigen*

HEPATITIS B, see *Australian Antigen*

HEPATITIS B SURFACE ANTIGEN, see *Australian Antigen*

HERPES

There are three different forms of herpes virus: herpes simplex (or herpes virus hominus) type I and type II, and herpes zoster. Herpes simplex type I causes the cold sores (fever blisters) that appear most commonly on the lips, in and around the mouth, and sometimes in the throat. Type II is usually limited to sores on the genital organs and is acquired primarily by sexual contact, but it can be transmitted to a baby during the birth process. Both types of herpes virus hominus can also cause meningitis and severe, even fatal encephalitis. The third form of herpes virus, herpes zoster, causes varicella (chicken pox) and shingles. Usually scrapings from a lesion are examined for specific identification; sometimes the material from the sore is injected into an animal for a more positive diagnosis.

When performed: When a patient has repeated attacks of cold sores or blisterlike sores around the genitals; when there is suspicion of shingles.

Normal values: Normally herpes virus is not found in body lesions. A person who has repeated bouts of cold sores, however, will carry herpes virus hominus type I for many years (sometimes for life), whether the sores are present or not.

Abnormal values: The presence of any of the three types of herpes virus is considered abnormal.

HETEROPHILE AGGLUTINATION, see *Agglutination*

HETEROPHILE ANTIBODY, see *Mononucleosis*

HETEROTROPIA, see *Strabismus*

HGH, see *Growth Hormone*

HIAA, see *Serotonin*

HIGH BLOOD PRESSURE, see *Blood Pressure*

HIGH-DENSITY LIPOPROTEIN, see *Cholesterol*; *Lipoproteins*

HINTON, see *Syphilis*

HIRSCHBERG, see *Strabismus*

HISTAMINE ACID, see *Gastric Analysis*

HISTOPLASMOSIS, see *Agglutination*

HIVES, see *Tartrazine Sensitivity*

HL-A ANTIGEN

Some white blood cells (leukocytes) and platelets contain antigens (disease-causing material) that initiates the formation of antibodies (disease-fighting material). These antigens are called human leukocyte locus A, or HL-A antigens. (Originally only one antigen location was discovered on a gene and it was called A; since then additional HL-A antigens have been found on locations other than "A.") Antileukocytic antibodies can be tested for by **Agglutination** or **Complement Fixation,** or by combining the suspected blood serum with lymphocytes (a particular type of **white blood cell**) and noting if the lymphocytes are destroyed, indicating the presence of an HL-A antibody.

The test is also used to determine histocompatibility, or whether the cells of tissues and organs from one person will "take" when transplanted into another person. There are many different HL-A antigens (approaching 100 at present), and the closer the donor-recipient agreement of HL-As, the better the chance that a transplant will not be rejected.

When performed: Primarily prior to any organ transplant operation (kidney, heart, or skin grafting); prior to some blood transfusions; with undiagnosed high-fever illnesses, arthritis, and anemia; as part of the many **Disputed Parentage** tests (each person inherits four basic HL-A antigens).

Normal values: There are no specific normal values; either the various HL-A antigens are present or they are not.

Abnormal values: The greater the number of HL-A typing dissimilarities, the less the chance that an organ transplant will take or that a skin graft will heal properly.

Different HL-A antigens have been associated with certain diseases. HL-A B27 is found in almost all cases of ankylosing spondylitis (an arthritic condition primarily of the sacroiliac joint and the spine); Reiter's syndrome (a disease, primarily found in men, that is characterized by an infection of the urethra with a discharge from the penis and an infection of the eye and the joints); in certain forms of arthritis in children prior to adolescence; and in a particular form of joint pain that occurs along with an infection of the bowels. A positive HL-A B27 is rarely found with true rheumatic disease. HL-A B13 and HL-A B17 (and occasionally HL-A B27) are usually found in patients with the arthritis of psoriasis. HL-A B7 is increased in patients with pernicious anemia. HL-A A2 is increased in patients with myasthenia gravis.

HOLTER MONITORING, see *Electrocardiogram*

HOLTZMAN INKBLOT TECHNIQUE, see *Rorschach*

HOMATROPINE, see *Tonometry*

HOMOCYSTINURIA, see *Aminoaciduria*

HOMOVANILLIC ACID, see *Catecholamines*

HOT CALORIC, see *Caloric*

HPL, see *Placental Lactogen*

HRR, see *Color Blindness*

HUMAN CHORIONIC SOMATOMAMMOTROPHIN, see *Placental Lactogen*

HUMAN GROWTH HORMONE, see *Growth Hormone*

HUMAN LEUKOCYTE LOCUS A, see *HL-A Antigen*

HUMAN PLACENTAL LACTOGEN, see *Placental Lactogen*

HVA, see *Catecholamines*

HYDROCHLORIC ACID, see *Gastric Analysis*

HYDROGEN ION CONTENT, see *pH*

HYDROXYBUTYRIC DEHYDROGENASE (HBD)

Alpha-hydroxybutyric dehydrogenase (HBD) is one of the many enzymes that appear in increased amounts in the serum subsequent to tissue damage. The HBD test is similar to the **Lactic Dehydrogenase** test in that it is supposed to be specific in diagnosing a heart attack, although the enzyme also increases slightly with liver disease, leukemia, and some cancers. It usually shows an abnormal rise within 12 hours after a heart attack and persists in an elevated state for up to a month. Blood is taken from a vein and the serum is tested.

When performed: Primarily as a confirmatory measure when a heart attack is suspected.

Normal values: Levels of 150 to 300 units per ml are considered normal.

Abnormal values: Levels usually rise to over 300 units per ml within 24 hours after a heart attack, reaching a peak, sometimes to 1,000 units per ml, in three days and then returning to normal during the next three weeks.

HYDROXYPROLINE

Hydroxyproline is an amino acid (one of the basic buildingblocks of proteins). It is unique in that it exists mostly in collagen, a substance found in bone and in slightly smaller amounts in the skin. While hydroxyproline levels are primarily an indication of a bone condition or bone disease, the test is also to search for certain inherited conditions. Although hydroxyproline can be found in the blood, the test is most often performed on urine.

When performed: When defects of bone metabolism are suspected (usually increased production or increased reabsorption of bone substance); after bone fractures; to follow the treatment of Paget's disease (an inflammation of the bones that causes deformation and bowing of arm and leg bones); to help diagnose rickets (vitamin D deficiency) and to follow the results of treatment; to aid in the diagnosis of certain inherited conditions such as Marfan's syndrome (a disease whose major feature is abnormally long bones).

Normal values: Total hydroxyproline levels range from 10 to 75 mg in a 24-hour specimen of urine.

Abnormal values: Increased amounts of hydroxyproline in the urine are found in most conditions where excessive bone structure is being made or repaired (fractures in children during normal growth, Marfan's syndrome, Paget's disease, and certain hormone problems). A decrease in hydroxyproline levels during treatment for certain bone diseases indicates successful therapy.

HYDROXYTRYPTAMINE, see *Serotonin*

HYPERGLYCEMIA, see *Glucose*

HYPERHIDROSIS, see *Sweat*

HYPERLIPIDEMIA, see *Lipids*

HYPERMETROPIA, see *Visual Acuity*

HYPEROPIA, see *Visual Acuity*

HYPEROXALURIA, see *Oxalate*

HYPERTENSION, see *Blood Pressure*

HYPNOTIC DRUG, see *Barbiturates*

HYPOGLYCEMIA, see *Glucose*

HYPOGONADISM, see *Testis Function*

HYSTEROSALPINGOGRAPHY, see *Radiography*

HYSTEROSCOPY, see *Endoscopy*

ICD, see *Isocitric Dehydrogenase*

ICG, see *Bromsulphalein*

ICTERUS INDEX

Icterus means jaundice. The icterus index measures the color of the blood serum as a gauge of its **Bilirubin** (yellow-brown bile pigment) content. Blood is drawn from a vein and the serum is compared with a standard solution of a normal serum color; the index is comparative density. While this test is considered outmoded by many physicians, it is still being performed; in most cases direct bilirubin is used as a more specific measurement.

When performed: When there is enlarged liver, tender liver, or a suggestion of jaundice of skin or eyes.

Normal values: An index of 3 to 5 is considered normal.

Abnormal values: An elevated index, between 6 and 15, indicates latent jaundice (jaundice that may not be apparent by examining skin or eyes) as with early hepatitis. An index above 15 indicates clinical jaundice, and indicates a non-specific form of liver and/or gall bladder disease. An index below 3 indicates decreased bilirubin, as in malaria and anemias.

ILLEGITIMACY, see *Disputed Parentage*

IMMUNE BODIES, see *Antinuclear Antibodies*

IMMUNITY, see *Immunoglobulin*

IMMUNOGLOBULIN (Ig)

Immunoglobulins (Ig) are the blood protein antibody particles (gamma globulins) of the body. They react with, protect against, and help destroy antigens, which can cause illness. An antigen may be a microorganism (bacteria, virus, fungus), a chemical, or a toxin given off by an invading microorganism. Usually antibodies are specific; that is, they react only to a particular disease-causing substance (either a new substance or one that has previously attacked the body). Antibodies come from lymphocyte (white blood) cells.

Five major immunoglobulins can be tested for in the blood (a sixth disappears after birth); they are known by letters of the alphabet. IgG (immunoglobulin G), the most abundant type, responds to any foreign-body invasion and can also cause Rh anemia problems. IgA protects against virus and bacterial infections and can cause transfusion reactions; IgM is another response to infection; it also reacts to arthritis and is the primary complement antibody (see **Complement Fixation**); IgE is involved in allergic reactions such as asthma, hay fever, and skin rashes (see **RAST**; **Skin Reaction**); IgD can be isolated, but its action is still not understood.

The presence of immunoglobulin is the basis on which **Agglutination** tests determine specific diseases. Immunoglobulins are measured individually primarily for purposes of research; they can, however, confirm diagnostic suspicions. Blood is taken from a vein and the serum is tested. Immunoglobulins are also tested in spinal fluid.

When performed: When excessive gamma globulins (hypergammaglobulinemia) are found, as with leukemias, certain cancers, kidney problems, parasitic infections, and chronic infections; after surgery for cancer as a guide to progress.

Normal values: Normal serum levels for the five major immunoglobulins are as follows:

IgG:	500 to 2,000 mg per 100 ml
IgA:	50 to 400 mg per 100 ml
IgM:	50 to 200 mg per 100 ml
IgE:	0.01 to 0.10 mg per 100 ml
IgD:	0.5 to 5 mg per 100 ml

Abnormal values: Immunoglobulins are increased as a result of infection, allergy, and various autoimmune conditions in which the body in essence turns on itself and causes illness (as in systemic lupus erythematosus). After cancer surgery, an increase in immunoglobulins is usually a good prognostic sign. Immunoglobulins may be decreased with certain leukemias, cancers, and other conditions where immunity is lacking.

Note: Cryoglobulins are immunoglobulins that precipitate only in cold temperatures and are present primarily with blood vessel diseases.

IMPEDENCE PLETHYSMOGRAPHY, see *Plethysmography*

IMPOTENCE (Male)

Although most male impotence (inability to achieve an erection of the penis) is thought to be of a psychological nature, in a substantial number of instances the problem has an organic (physical) basis or is caused by taking certain drugs. Alcohol, many medicines that treat high blood pressure, many tranquilizers, and most hormones can cause impotence and/or loss of libido. Specific drugs reported to cause loss of sexual desire and impotence in men and frigidity in women include guanethidine (Ismelin), methyldopa, clonidine (Catapres), rauwolfia and reserpine compounds, phentolamine, tolazoline, phenoxybenamine, propranolol (Inderol), Aldactone, and thiazide diuretics (for treating blood pressure and circulatory problems); the benzodiazepines and other minor tranquilizers such as Dalmane, Librium, Valium, Serax, and Tranxene; the phenothiazines and other major tranquilizers such as Mellaril; monoamine oxidase inhibitors, tricyclic drugs, and lithium (for treating depression); anticholinergic drugs (for treating and relaxing irritable stomach, bladder, and bowel as well as for glaucoma and parkinsonism); certain antibiotic drugs such as nitrofurantoin and ethionamide and parasite-killing drugs such as thiabendazole; drugs used to attack cancer cells; almost all narcotics; marijuana; and methadone.

It is extremely difficult to differentiate between psychological and physical causes of impotence. One specific test requires the patient to spend at least three consecutive nights in a laboratory that has facilities for measuring REM (rapid eye movement) levels of sleep (the deepest stage) as well as nocturnal penile tumescence (swelling). Electrodes are placed on the head and are attached to silicone rings around the penis; measurements are made throughout the night during sleep. (See also **Plethysmography** and **Thermography**.)

When performed: When impotence cannot be diagnosed; prior to surgical penile prosthesis implant insertion; following head, spinal cord, or back injuries.

Normal values: Most men have several penile erections during the night when in deep stages of sleep, especially while dreaming. Such a response indicates no physical pathology or disease as a cause of impotence.

Abnormal values: Failure to show any penile response after three days of testing indicates some physical basis for impotence. Normally the number of nocturnal sleeping erections decreases in men over 50, but total absence indicates a nerve, blood vessel, or spinal cord problem.

INCOMPATIBLE TRANSFUSION, see *Typing and Cross-Matching*

INDIRECT BILIRUBIN, see *Bilirubin*

INDOCYANINE GREEN, see *Bromsulphalein*

INFECTION, see *Agglutination, Complement Fixation*

INFECTIOUS MONONUCLEOSIS, see *Mononucleosis*

INFLUENZA, see *Complement Fixation*

INKBLOT, see *Rorschach*

INSECTICIDE POISONING, see *Cholinesterase*

INSULIN

Direct measurement of insulin in the blood is primarily an indication of the ability of the pancreas to secrete this hormone (the stomach can also secrete a very small amount) in response to carbohydrate foods, certain amino and fatty acids, and certain other hormones and drugs.

The patient is asked to fast for 12 hours before the test. Blood is taken from a vein and the serum is tested. At times, the patient is then given a measured amount of glucose (sugar) and the blood insulin is measured every half-hour for three to four hours. The test cannot be performed on a patient taking insulin injections.

When performed: When diabetes is suspected; when physical growth problems are evident; as an indication of whether certain oral antidiabetic drugs will work; when pancreatic disease, especially tumor, is suspected.

Normal values: After a 12-hour fast, the amount of serum insulin normally measures from 5 to 30 μU per ml. After glucose is given, blood insulin levels usually rise to more than 200 μU per ml within an hour and return to normal after four hours.

Abnormal values: Insulin levels are increased with an insulinoma (a tumor of insulin-producing cells), obesity, liver disease, and acromegaly (abnormally enlarged bones). Certain hormone drugs will also raise insulin levels. Insulin is lower than normal with diabetes, following surgery, after a heart attack, and when certain other hormones are absent from the body. Patients under emotional stress will also have reduced amounts of insulin secretion.

INSULIN ACIDITY, see *Gastric Analysis*

INSULIN-CORTISOL SECRETION, see *Cortisol*

INSULIN PRODUCTION, see *C-Peptide*

INTELLIGENCE QUOTIENT (IQ)

The first mass use of the intelligence test was in France around 1900 as part of an effort by the government to distinguish children who could benefit from going to school from those who were considered too dull for an education. Today, there is little agreement on a universal definition of intelligence. It is generally recognized as an ability to make use of learning, reasoning, and memory in problem solving.

Most intelligence tests measure an individual's ability to learn in comparison with the general population. The IQ (intelligence quotient) is expressed by dividing the mental age (as determined in the test) by the chronological age (the actual age in years and months) and then multiplying the result by 100. Thus a ten-year-old with average mental ability for that age would have an IQ of $10/10 \times 100 = 100$.

Numerous forms of IQ tests are in use today. The Stanford-Binet relies heavily on verbal ability in its scoring and is therefore considered deficient in recognizing an individual's strengths and special abilities. The Wechsler Intelligence Scale for Children (WISC) and the Wechsler Adult Intelligence Scale

(WAIS) include both verbal and physical performance tests; it is felt that the combined verbal and performance scores offer a better individual profile than verbal scores alone. Performance measurements are especially valuable in testing the handicapped, young children, and people of foreign background with a limited knowledge of the language of the test. Performance tests are considered better than verbal tests as predictors of adjustment, while verbal tests are considered better predictors of educational achievement.

Group intelligence tests used in schools and the military are not considered to yield results as accurate as individual tests. The group tests determine whether a subject is performing up to ability and is capable of taking on more advanced work. A few of the many group tests include the Army General Classification Test, the Otis Self-Administering Test of Mental Ability, the Kuhlmann-Anderson Intelligence Tests, and the Terman-McNemar Test of Mental Ability.

When performed: To assess the mental skills and learning ability of different individuals or groups; to discern dementia (physically caused mental deterioration).

Normal values: In general, IQ scores of 90 to 110 are considered average; a score of 140 or more is referred to as the genius level. On the average, the Wechsler scale results are about 7 points below the Stanford-Binet score. Other tests may vary slightly in scoring.

Abnormal values: IQ scores of 20 to 35 are considered indicative of severe mental retardation; 36 to 51, of moderate mental retardation; 52 to 67, of mild mental retardation; and 68 to 83, of borderline mental retardation. A person with a definite psychosis will have spotty responses (missing simple questions yet answering difficult ones). Senility due to arteriosclerosis will give a lowered score.

Note: The results of any type of IQ test should be evaluated with caution, especially if only one test is performed. In certain cases the courts have held that an error in IQ reporting, causing a person embarrassment or difficulty, may be compensated by a monetary award.

INTESTINAL ABSORPTION, see *Xylose Tolerance*

INTRACUTANEOUS, see *Skin Reaction*

INTRADERMAL, see *Skin Reaction*

INTRAOCULAR PRESSURE, see *Tonometry*

INTRATHECAL SCAN, see *Nuclear Scanning*

INTRINSIC FACTOR, see *Schilling*

INULIN CLEARANCE, see *Creatinine*

IODINE, see *Thyroid Function*

IQ, see *Intelligence Quotient*

IRON

While the iron test is performed primarily to measure the amount of iron in the body, it is more a measure of the total iron-binding capacity, or the iron's availability to pick up oxygen from the lungs and deliver it to body tissues. Body iron is affected by pregnancy, blood loss, hemoglobin destruction, anemia, deficient iron in the diet, and poor intestinal absorption of iron even when dietary amounts are adequate. An average, balanced diet supplies about 10 mg of iron each day, but no more than 10% of that iron is normally absorbed by the intestines to be utilized. At the same time, the body loses about 1 mg of iron a day (through urine, feces, and sweat). Fortunately, the body usually has a large store of excess iron. Blood is collected from a vein and either the serum or plasma is tested. When repeated iron tests are performed, it is essential that the blood samples be taken at the same time of the day. Iron values are usually highest in the morning, after sleep, and may be half the morning's value by evening. These findings are reversed for people who work nights and sleep days.

Other measures of blood and body iron are the serum iron-binding capacity (transferrin), or the specific amount of iron that can be carried in plasma; and the ferritin level, or the amount of iron stored in the body (primarily in the bone marrow). A patient can have a normal amount of iron, but that iron may not carry and deliver a sufficient amount of oxygen to the tissues.

When performed: In searching for the specific cause of an anemia; when there is unexplained weakness and persistent tiredness; when the patient has a swollen, smooth, painful tongue.

Normal values: Iron levels generally range from 75 to 175 mcg per 100 ml of serum. Normal values may vary depending on the laboratory's technique. The values may be slightly lower in women and children. Total iron-binding capacity ranges from 200 to 400 mcg per 100 ml. Serum ferritin ranges from 200 to 400 ng per 100 ml.

Abnormal values: Low blood values are found with anemia, infections, cancers, and pruritis (itching skin); after surgery; and in patients taking steroid drugs. Oral contraceptives, estrogens, or excessive dietary iron intake especially from iron-fortified foods may give elevated values. Extremely high levels of iron and iron-binding capacity are found with hemochromatosis, an inherited intestinal iron absorption disease that can cause sufficient iron accumulation in the body so as to be fatal before the age of 30. Total iron-binding capacity is usually increased only with an iron deficiency anemia; it is normal or decreased with other anemias. Total iron-binding capacity and transferrin may be artificially increased by birth control pills or other female hormones. Decreased ferritin is found with iron deficiency but not with anemia of infection; increased ferritin is found with excessive iron intake.

IRON-BINDING CAPACITY, see *Iron*

ISHIHARA, see *Color Blindness*

ISOCITRIC DEHYDROGENASE

Testing for isocitric dehydrogenase (an enzyme found mostly in the liver) is particularly valuable in detecting and distinguishing liver disease. It can also reflect problems with the placenta during pregnancy. Most recently it has been used to screen blood donors in order to eliminate the possibility of transmitting infectious hepatitis by blood transfusions. Blood is taken from a vein and the serum is tested.

When performed: Primarily with suspected liver disease, especially to help differentiate disease that originates within the liver cells from disease that originates outside the liver (most commonly from the bile ducts) but that still reflects itself as liver pathology; when cancer of the liver, usually metastatic (migrated from another source), is suspected; during pregnancy as an indication of placenta problems.

Normal values: Normal levels range from 50 to 300 units per ml.

Abnormal values: Increased levels indicate liver disease, especially hepatitis or cancer. If a pregnant woman has no liver problem, an increase is a warning that something is wrong with the placenta.

ISOENZYMES, see *Creatine Phosphokinase, Glutamic Oxalacetic Transaminase, Lactic Dehydrogenase*

ISOPROPYL ALCOHOL, see *Methanol*

IVC, see *Radiography*

IVP, see *Radiography*

IVY BLEEDING TIME, see *Bleeding and Clotting Time*

JENKINS ACTIVITY SURVEY

Of the many factors being studied as potential indicators of increased risk of heart disease, especially heart attack, the psychological makeup of an individual is among those in the forefront. Studies of individual behavior patterns—particularly a person's competitiveness in activities such as employment, his ambitions, his attitudes toward time (sense of urgency), and even the way he speaks—have indicated two basic personality types in relation to heart disease risk. Type A is aggressive, highly competitive, always striving to get ahead, and extremely time-conscious. Type B is just the opposite: outwardly relaxed and seldom impatient. The Type B personality takes ample time for recreational activities and speaks more slowly and evenly than his Type A counterpart.

Doctors can sometimes determine a personality type by speaking with a patient over a period of time and noting the nature of the patient's responses (especially the reaction to feigned hostility). The Jenkins Activity Survey provides a more standardized format for evaluating the coronary-prone personality. The test was first employed in 1965; since that time nearly 100,000 people (primarily men) have taken it, demonstrating by the results that those who score as Type A have from five to eight times as many heart attacks as those who score as Type B.

The survey comprises 61 multiple-choice questions, which the patient completes in private. A sample question is: "Nowadays do you consider yourself to be (1) definitely hard-driving and competitive, (2) probably hard-driving and competitive, (3) probably relaxed and easygoing, or (4) definitely relaxed and easygoing?" The first answer indicates Type A; the second answer could be either Type A or Type B; the third answer is Type B; the fourth answer is rare.

There are now more than a dozen similar tests, including "structured" interviews as well as variations on the specific business and personal activities used to measure alleged coronary-prone behavior (socioeconomic status, social mobility, cultural background, and even smoking are predominant factors in some of the tests). Before the test is conducted, subjects should be told to view the questions as a measure of their attitudes and life ambitions rather than solely as a survey of heart disease potential.

When performed: The survey is used primarily as a screening device to determine Type A or Type B personality traits, with particular association to heart disease. The test may be performed on healthy individuals and used as a future study or research index, or it may be performed on patients with known heart disease to help ascertain the test's validity. It may also be used to show a patient facets of his nature that he may be unaware of so he can better understand stress-inducing circumstances.

Normal values: While there are no normal values for such a test, obviously the more Type B answers, the less the individual reacts to stress in a supposedly unhealthy manner.

Abnormal values: Assuming the validity of the test in helping to detect coronary-prone individuals, the more Type A answers a person gives, the greater the risk of heart disease.

JOINT ARTHROGRAPHY, see *Radiography*

JOINT FLUID, see *Synovial Fluid*

JOINT FLUID CULTURE, see *Culture*

JUGULAR VEIN PULSE, see *Pulse Analysis*

KAHN, see *Syphilis*

KAOLIN-CEPHALIN CLOTTING TIME, see *Partial Thromboplastin Time*

KARYOTYPING, see *Amniocentesis*

KATAYAMA, see *Hemoglobin*

KETONES (Ketone Bodies)

Ketones (two different acids and acetone) are produced in the body when glycogen (a form of carbohydrate) is not available to be utilized for energy. The body then draws upon its fat deposits, which are improperly oxidized and which then produce excessive amounts of ketones in both the blood and the urine. When insulin is absent or not immediately available to metabolize carbohydrates (as in diabetes), fats will be burned for body energy, creating more ketones than the body can utilize. Blood plasma from a vein is examined; urine is usually examined at the same time.

When performed: Especially when a patient is in a coma; to diagnose diabetic acidosis; when there is a question of toxemia in pregnancy; with hyperthyroidism and other metabolic abnormalities.

Since ketones are a "desirable" side effect of the no (or very low) carbohydrate, high protein and fat weight-loss diet, they are constantly tested for in the urine by the dieter as an indication that excessive body fats are being metabolized.

Normal values: Ketones are not usually detected in the blood; however, up to 3 mg per 100 ml is considered within normal limits. There are very few ketones in the urine (125 mg per 24-hour sample, an amount that would not be detected by the usual urine acetone tests).

Abnormal values: More than 3 mg per 100 ml of serum is considered excessive. In diabetic acidosis, levels over 100 mg per 100 ml may be reached. Excessive ketones are found in the blood and urine in metabolic disorders, in starvation, and after a few days on a no-carbohydrate diet. They are also found in the urine with an inherited condition called maple syrup urine disease (the urine smells like fresh maple syrup) and with another inherited condition called renal glycosuria (the kidneys excrete sugar even though the blood sugar is normal). There may be a false elevation of ketones after administration of the **Bromsulphalein** test.

KETOSTEROIDS, see *Cortisol*

KIDNEY SCAN, see *Nuclear Scanning*

KIDNEY STONE, see *Urinary Tract Calculus*

KINETOCARDIOGRAM, see *Apexcardiogram*

KISSING DISEASE, see *Mononucleosis*

KLINE, see *Syphilis*

KNEE ARTHROGRAPHY, see *Radiography*

KNEE ENDOSCOPY, see *Endoscopy*

KNEE JERK, see *Reflex*

KOLMER, see *Syphilis*

KUHLMANN-ANDERSON, see *Intelligence Quotient*

KVEIM

The Kveim test is a special skin test to aid in diagnosing sarcoidosis (Boeck's sarcoid disease), a condition in which the lymph glands enlarge and fibrous nodules appear in the chest and other body areas. Sarcoidosis is often mistaken for tuberculosis; the Kveim test helps differentiate the two conditions.

The exact cause of sarcoidosis is not known, but it is believed to be a virus disease. It is found mostly in young adults living in the South and in blacks far more than in whites. A tiny amount of known sarcoid tissue is injected into the skin; the injection site is watched for a reaction over the next six to eight weeks.

When performed: When sarcoidosis or tuberculosis is suspected, usually after an abnormal chest X-ray; to prevent the need for a surgical procedure to enter the chest and obtain a nodule for **Biopsy**; with a chronic cough that cannot easily be diagnosed.

Normal values: There should be no reaction at the site of injection after eight weeks.

Abnormal values: In patients with sarcoidosis, a small growth appears at the injection site, usually within six weeks; when that growth is examined under the microscope, specific sarcoid granulomas are seen. While the test is considered accurate in nearly 90% of cases of sarcoidosis, it can on occasion be positive with other conditions.

LACRIMAL, see *Schirmer's*

LACTIC ACID

Lactic acid is an end product of sugar metabolism. When the body increases lactic acid production or fails to excrete lactic acid, the condition is called lactic acidosis (usually a complication of kidney, heart, or liver disease).

Lactic acidosis is characterized by a marked "anion gap." Normally the amount of sodium plus the amount of potassium in the blood (anion group) equals the total amount of chloride and bicarbonate in the blood (cation group). When the difference between the two groups is greater than 30 (that is, when the cation group is decreased), an anion gap exists and is an ominous sign of lactic acidosis. Blood is taken from a vein and the whole blood is tested.

When performed: When there is rapid deep breathing, somnolence, stupor, or coma; when metabolic acidosis is suspected; when an anion gap exists.

Normal values: Lactic acid levels from 5 to 20 mg per 100 ml.

Abnormal values: Elevated blood lactic acid is indicative of lactic acidosis. It can also result from exercise, anemia, leukemias, diabetes mellitus, the taking of certain drugs such as epinephrine for asthma or phenformin for diabetes, and salicylate (aspirin) intoxication.

LACTIC ACID DEHYDROGENASE, see *Lactic Dehydrogenase*

LACTIC DEHYDROGENASE (LDH)

Serum lactic dehydrogenase (LDH) is an enzyme found in many body organs and in red blood cells, which when damaged or diseased release that enzyme into the blood serum. LDH acts as a catalyst in carbohydrate metabolism. There are five different forms (isoenzymes) of LDH, concentrated in varying amounts in such organs as the heart and liver and in the muscles.

Most commonly the total LDH is measured; occasionally the different forms of LDH are tested to help ascertain the location and sometimes the extent of body damage. Blood is taken from a vein and the serum is examined. LDH is also measured in spinal fluid, in pleural (lung) fluid, and in the urine, where it is sometimes used as a screening test for kidney and bladder cancer.

When performed: When there is suspicion of a heart attack or cancer; to diagnose anemia; to aid in determining if a mother is carrying a child with an Rh problem; to distinguish hepatitis from other liver diseases; to aid in the diagnosis of pulmonary embolism.

Normal values: Normal LDH levels range from 200 to 600 units per ml of serum or up to 250 IU. Because different laboratories use so many different methods for testing, normal values may vary greatly.

Abnormal values: Lower than normal values of LDH may be found after excessive X-ray exposure. Increased values are found after a heart attack. LDH levels do not become elevated as rapidly as certain other enzymes tested for when heart disease is suspected (see **Creatinine Phosphokinase** and **Glutamic Oxalacetic Transaminase**). When elevated, LDH levels persist much longer. Extremely high values of LDH are found with hepatitis, infectious mononucleosis, and anemias caused by deficiencies of vitamin B_{12} or folic acid. Elevated LDH levels are also seen with leukemia and other cancers, but the test is not specific enough to be the sole basis for diagnosis.

Elevated levels of certain isoenzymes of LDH indicate heart disease; others point to liver problems and are more disease-specific. When total LDH levels are elevated, an LDH heat fractionization test is sometimes performed. After LDH is subjected to high heat, only the heart-produced isoenzymes remain, helping to pinpoint the diagnosis.

LDH levels are increased in the spinal fluid following a stroke and with meningitis. In chest conditions that cause the surface of the lungs to give off fluid (pleurisy), the fluid has high LDH levels. With a urinary tract infection or a growth anywhere from the kidney to the bladder, urine LDH levels are elevated.

LACTOGENIC HORMONE, see *Prolactin*

LACTOSE TOLERANCE

Lactose is a type of sugar found only in milk. Some people do not have sufficient lactase (an enzyme) to break down milk sugar; as a result, they have many different symptoms (mostly gastrointestinal cramps and bloating) after drinking milk or eating milk products. Because lactose is broken down in the making of cheese, this food is usually tolerated by patients with milk intolerance. Intolerance to milk sugar is not an allergy, and the symptoms are not the same as an allergic reaction to milk protein. Usually the symptoms are as a result of ingesting an increased quantity of milk (people without lactase can usually drink milk or cream in coffee or on cereal). The condition is found most commonly in Orientals, Arabs, blacks, Italians, and Ashkenazi Jews.

In the lactose tolerance test, a patient is given a measured amount of a lactose solution to drink after a fasting blood sugar test (see **Glucose**) has been performed. An hour or two later another blood sugar test is performed.

When performed: When a patient complains of persistent abdominal or gas pains, especially if the patient's intake of milk has increased.

Normal values: Blood sugar rather than lactose itself is measured. Normally after a patient drinks the lactose solution, the blood sugar will rise at least 40 mg per 100 ml within an hour or two.

Abnormal values: Failure of the blood sugar to rise more than 20 mg per 100 ml after drinking the lactose solution is indicative of lactose intolerance. Elderly patients with certain bone diseases may also show an abnormal result, as will some patients who have recently had gastrointestinal surgery or who have an "irritable" bowel.

LANGUAGE FUNCTION

Defects in language function (aphasia) may be of an expressive nature (difficulty in planning, coordinating, and using speech), a receptive nature (unable to understand what is said), or amnesic (unable to remember sounds). Testing for the type of aphasia helps locate the exact area of brain disease. The patient is asked to recite the alphabet, count forward and backward, spell words, and read a poem. Next, the patient is asked to repeat particular phrases such as Methodist Episcopal and the Peter Piper doggerel. Spoken and written commands such as "button your vest," or "hold out your hand and spread your fingers" are given and the response noted. Finally, the patient is asked to name familiar sounds such as the mewing of a cat, the ticking of a watch, and running water. There are many other tests for aphasia; the specific type depends on the physician's preference. All language function evaluations must take into account the patient's educational experience.

When performed: Whenever brain disease is suspected; in stroke; in certain infectious diseases that affect the brain such as syphilis.

Normal values: Normal patients have no difficulty speaking and understanding the language.

Abnormal values: Speech impairment almost always indicates disease of the left side of the brain. With receptive types of aphasia, the pathology is usually in the temporal (side) area; amnesic aphasia suggests frontal area brain disease; patients with expressive aphasia often accompanied by the inability to write out a word with eyes closed, signifies damage in the brain cortex (where motion and purposeful activity are controlled). Inability to know left from right, when accompanied by disturbed language function, may reflect brain disease.

Note: Some doctors feel there is no such thing as "baby talk"; failure of an adult to use proper sounds (phonetics) is usually indicative of a disability such as minimal brain dysfunction. Persistent "baby talk" can also indicate abnormal anxiety and other mental health problems.

LAP, see *Leucine Aminopeptidase*

LAPAROSCOPY, see *Endoscopy*

LATEX AGGLUTINATION, see *Agglutination*

LATEX FIXATION, see *Agglutination*

LATS, see *Thyroid Function*

LDH, see *Lactic Dehydrogenase*

LEAD

Lead is a trace element (only a trace is normally found in the body) that can produce a toxic reaction (plumbism) when sufficient amounts enter the body. At one time most paint had a lead base. Infants who chewed on toys or cribs painted with lead-based paint were apt to suffer lead poisoning. Today most paints are lead-free; however, old walls, furniture, and toys that have been painted over may still have lead paint underneath, posing a hazard if the paint chips or peels. Lead poisoning can also occur in people whose occupation puts them in contact with lead and people who are exposed to heavy vehicular traffic (policemen).

Whole blood, urine, and body tissues such as liver, bone, and hair may be examined. The urine may also be examined for delta aminolevulinic acid (ALA) and coproporphyrin as a screening test for those whose jobs involve contact with lead.

When performed: To aid in the diagnosis of lead poisoning; in children with pica (the regular eating of dirt and other foreign material).

Normal values: Normally traces of lead up to 40 mcg per 100 ml may be found in the blood. Urine lead should not exceed 100 mcg per 24-hour sample. Hair should show lead levels below 20 mcg per gram.

Abnormal values: Levels over 40 mcg per 100 ml of whole blood or over 100 mcg in a 24-hour urine specimen are indicative of lead intoxication. More than 50 mcg per gram of hair reveals plumbism.

LEARNING ABILITY NECK REFLEX, see *Reflex*

LE CELL, see *Antinuclear Antibodies*

LEE-WHITE COAGULATION, see *Bleeding and Clotting Time*

LEFT VENTRICULAR EJECTION TIME, see *Systolic Time Intervals*

LEUCINE AMINOPEPTIDASE

Leucine aminopeptidase (LAP) is an enzyme produced by the liver, the pancreas, and the small intestine. LAP tests are performed when various other enzyme tests seem to conflict, especially in diagnosing liver disease and in determining whether elevated levels of **Alkaline Phosphatase** are caused by liver problems as opposed to bone disease. Blood is taken from a vein and the serum is tested.

When performed: Primarily to distinguish bile duct obstruction from liver cell disease.

Normal values: Depending on the method used by various laboratories, normal values can differ; one measure is from 5 to 25 standard units per ml.

Abnormal values: LAP is increased when the bile ducts are obstructed (causing liver disease); it is normal or lower than normal when liver pathology comes from within the liver cells.

LEUKOCYTE, see *White Blood Cell*

LEUKOCYTE ANTIBODY, see *HL-A Antigen*

LEUKOCYTE DIFFERENTIAL, see *Blood Cell Differential*

LEWIS, see *Cystometry*

LIMULUS ASSAY, see *Synovial Fluid*

LIPASE

Lipase, an enzyme secreted by the pancreas, helps to break down triglyceride fats so they can be utilized by the body. In the blood lipase levels usually parallel those of **Amylase** (another fat-splitting enzyme produced by the pancreas), and the two are generally tested together. Blood is drawn from a vein and the serum is examined.

When performed: When disease of the pancreas is suspected and a definite diagnosis is not certain.

Normal values: Normal levels of lipase range from 0.2 units to 1.5 units per ml.

Abnormal values: Serum lipase levels are elevated in pancreatitis (but not as much as amylase levels), in cancer of the pancreas and certain intestinal ulcers, and in patients using opiate drugs (morphine, codeine).

LIPIDS

The total lipids test includes the measurement of the three major lipids (fats) in blood serum: cholesterol (an alcohol, not a true fat, yet still so categorized medically), triglycerides, and phospholipids. The test also includes the free fatty acids and other fats, but at present these have no diagnostic significance. Phospholipids (e.g., lecithin) also offer little diagnostic information, but a few physicians employ the phospholipid/cholesterol ratio as an experimental indication of atherosclerosis (see **Cholesterol**).

Triglycerides comprise the greatest amount (by weight) of lipids in the blood as well as in the foods we eat and are considered true fats (olive oil is made up in large part of triglycerides). While triglycerides come primarily from fats in the diet, like cholesterol they can also be manufactured by the liver. Triglycerides are the blood fats that reflect light; thus, in samples taken after a fatty meal or when there is some metabolic defect, they may be seen as a turbid layer in a test tube of serum that has been left standing. Alcohol and carbohydrates, more than fatty foods, cause a great increase in blood triglyceride levels.

The triglyceride test may be performed independently, but it is commonly measured along with cholesterol. The two tests, along with observation of the serum after refrigeration overnight in a test tube, are considered together to arrive at a classification of hyperlipidemia when an excess of serum lipids exists. Lipidemia (the normal amounts of fat in the blood) is often confused with lipoproteinemia, which is another classification of the various densities of the protein molecules that attach themselves to and carry the lipids in the blood (see **Lipoproteins**).

Blood is taken from a vein and the serum or plasma is tested. For triglycerides, the patient should follow a normal diet for at least two weeks before the test and should then eat nothing for 14 hours before the blood is taken. Certain drugs such as hormones, steroids, birth control pills, and diuretics must not be taken for a month before the tests.

When performed: Blood lipids are measured to reflect familial (inherited) disorders of fat metabolism (not necessarily disease-producing); they can point to possible liver, kidney, and thyroid diseases, and at times signify bile tract obstruction; today, however, they are tested mostly as an experimental indication of atherosclerosis.

Normal values: Total lipids usually range from 400 to 1,000 mg per 100 ml (they are normally increased after a meal containing fat). Triglycerides range from 30 to 145 mg per 100 ml; phospholipids, from 125 to 350 mg per 100 ml; the phospholipid/cholesterol ratio, from 0.7 to 1.8.

Abnormal values: There is as yet no scientific agreement on the relative merits of serum lipid measurements for the prognosis of heart and artery disease. Thus, while six varieties of hyperlipidemia (elevated serum lipid levels) have been postulated as a guide to the degree of risk for atherosclerosis, these hypothetical abnormalities are just that—hypothetical. The types are classified according to whether triglycerides, cholesterol, or both are elevated (along with the appearance of the plasma and the patient's symptoms, if any).

Type I, while very rare, shows only high triglycerides. Patients may suffer abdominal pain, but the risk of heart disease is thought to be low.

There are two kinds of type II: the most common, IIa, shows only an increased cholesterol level; IIb shows elevated cholesterol and triglycerides. Both are alleged to be indications of heart disease.

Type III, extremely rare, shows high cholesterol and triglyceride levels but also shows elevated glucose (sugar) levels. It too is alleged to be a warning sign of heart disease.

Type IV, similar to but more common than type III, shows only a marked triglyceride elevation.

Type V, rare, also shows only a triglyceride elevation and is believed to be a combination of types I and IV.

It has been postulated that the lower the phospholipid/cholesterol ratio (decreased phospholipids), the greater the possibility of atherosclerosis. Again, the reasoning behind the classification of lipids is to discover if there is a way to utilize such typing as a means of identifying those at risk for atherosclerosis.

LIPOPROTEINS

When **Lipids** (fat molecules) combine in the blood with protein molecules, they are called lipoproteins. Lipoproteins are classified according to their density: those with more fat and less protein have the least density (lightest weight); those with the least fat and the most protein have the highest density. Classifying the different lipoproteins is called phenotyping.

The lipoprotein containing the least amount of protein (1%), consists largely of triglycerides and is called a chylomicron. The very-low-density lipoproteins (VLDL), sometimes called pre-beta, contain more than half triglycerides as well as almost equal amounts of cholesterol and phospholipids and up to 10% proteins. The low-density lipoproteins (LDL), sometimes called beta, are nearly half cholesterol, with almost equal amounts of triglycerides and phospholipids along with 20% proteins. The high-density lipoproteins (HDL), sometimes called alpha, are composed mostly of proteins and phospholipids. The presence of increased amounts of high-density lipoproteins in the blood has been associated with a noticeable lack of heart and artery disease. Thus, in tests for **Cholesterol**, the amount of high-density lipoproteins is more important than simply total cholesterol alone. HDL levels are rarely influenced by the type of fat (saturated or polyunsaturated) a person eats; they are increased by exercise, weight loss, niacin (vitamin B_3), and moderate amounts of alcohol while decreased on a high carbohydrate diet.

The four different lipoproteins are also utilized in ascertaining the six types of hyperlipidemia (see **Lipids**). Type I shows almost all chylomicrons. Type II has two variations: IIa is mostly very-low-density lipoproteins; IIb is mostly both very-low-density lipoproteins and low-density lipoproteins. Type III shows abnormal low-density and very-low-density lipoproteins. Types IV and V show increased very-low-density lipoprotein. Type V also shows an increased amount of chylomicrons. The classifications are primarily measurements to see if predisposition to atherosclerosis (heart and artery disease) can someday be predicted. Blood is taken from a vein for testing.

When performed: To study and classify people with elevated lipids (cholesterol or triglycerides) as a possible aid in detecting patients with greater than average risk of heart and artery disease.

Normal values: There are, at this time, no definitive standards; the descriptions above give an indication of the usual composition of each lipid protein.

Abnormal values: The presence of excessive amounts of very-low-density lipoproteins is tentatively assumed to be a prognostic sign of atherosclerosis. In contrast, large amounts of high-density lipoproteins are believed to be a prognostic sign of some built-in protection against atherosclerosis.

LITHIUM

Lithium salts have been found to be effective in the treatment of manic-depressive illness—primarily to prevent and treat the mania, but occasionally to lessen the depression. Because of the toxic effects of lithium, patients who are on maintenance treatment must be monitored closely so that they can benefit from the drug with as few adverse effects as possible.

The blood level of lithium is tested the day after treatment starts. It is then tested three times a week until the proper maintenance level is established. Afterward it is tested monthly (sooner if symptoms appear). The patient must not take lithium for eight hours prior to the test. Blood is drawn from a vein and serum is examined.

When performed: To follow patients with manic-depressive disease who are being treated with lithium; to adjust the dosage of the drug as necessary.

Normal values: Normally there is no lithium in blood serum. A therapeutic blood level of lithium is considered to range from 0.5 to 1.5 mEq per liter. But even at the therapeutic level, the patient may have side effects, such as excessive thirst and urination, upset stomach, diarrhea, slight tremor, and increased white blood cell count.

Abnormal values: Blood levels of lithium over 1.5 mEq per liter are considered toxic. When there is a toxic amount of lithium in the blood, the patient may suffer from vomiting, muscle weakness, convulsions, leukocytosis, coma, and death (at 4 mEq per liter). Diuretics or a low-salt diet can cause an increased serum level of lithium.

LIVER ENZYME, see *Isocitric Dehydrogenase*

LIVER SCAN, see *Nuclear Scanning*

LOMBARD, see *Hearing Function*

LONG-ACTING THYROID STIMULATOR, see *Thyroid Function*

LOWER-BOWEL X-RAY, see *Radiography*

LOWER GI SERIES, see *Radiography*

LUMBAR PUNCTURE, see *Cerebrospinal Fluid*

LUNG, see *Pulmonary Function*

LUNG FLUID, see *Thoracentesis*

LUNG SCAN, see *Nuclear Scanning*

LUNG SECRETION, see *Sputum*

LUPUS ERYTHEMATOSUS (LE) CELL, see *Antinuclear Antibodies*

LYMPHANGIOGRAPHY, see *Radiography*

LYSOZYME

Lysozyme (or muramidase) is an enzyme that destroys certain bacteria, thus causing certain disease symptoms to subside. Lysozyme occurs naturally in some body fluids such as tears, saliva, serum, and breast milk; it is also found in some plants and in egg whites. The natural occurrence of lysozyme in mother's milk and saliva may account for the traditional beliefs that mother's milk helps protect babies from certain diseases, and that licking a wound is beneficial.

Lysozyme is also found in large amounts in monocytes (large white blood cells). Blood serum and/or urine is examined.

When performed: Lysozyme values are studied in patients with myelomonocytic and lymphocytic leukemia.

Normal values: In serum, 7 to 14 mcg per ml is a normal finding; in urine, 2 mcg per ml.

Abnormal values: Patients with myelomonocytic leukemia have elevated levels of lysozyme (as high as 230 mcg per ml). Patients with lymphocytic leukemia have decreased values (3 to 12 mcg per ml).

MACROGLOBULIN (Sia)

Macroglobulins are serum globulins (see **Albumin/Globulin**; **Immunoglobulin**) that are up to ten times heavier than the usual globulins. They are usually measured as an entity, but they can be broken down into separate parts; the largest portion (usually about two-thirds) is known as alpha-2. Macroglobulins comprise only about 5% of all globulins. In the Sia test, blood is taken from a vein for examination. The serum is diluted with water so that total macroglobulins are precipitated out of the solution.

When performed: Primarily when Waldenstrom's macroglobulinemia (a rare disease found most often in older men and characterized by anemia, enlarged liver and spleen, and hemorrhage) is suspected; when leukemia, certain cancers, and prolonged infections cannot be specifically diagnosed.

Normal values: Total macroglobulins average 0.4 g per 100 ml of serum (slightly higher in women). The alpha-2 portion ranges from 0.1 to 0.4 g per 100 ml.

Abnormal values: Increases of up to three times normal values (especially of alpha-2 macroglobulins) are found in Waldenstrom's macroglobulinemia. Total macroglobulins are increased in leukemia, multiple myeloma, certain cancers, and chronic infections. Increased macroglobulins can falsely increase the erythrocyte sedimentation rate. (See **Sedimentation Rate**).

MADDOX ROD, see *Strabismus*

MAGNESIUM

One of the most abundant minerals in the body, magnesium is found in all cells and is active in many biochemical processes, particularly in enzyme reactions. Magnesium is important to the regulation of the body's calcium supply and usage. A normal diet (particularly nuts and vegetables) affords the body about 0.5 g of magnesium every day. Blood is collected from a vein and serum is examined.

When performed: The test is performed whenever patients exhibit symptoms such as twitching and quivering muscles, irritability, and weakness. It is also used to determine whether these symptoms are caused by lowered calcium levels rather than by lowered magnesium levels. Low magnesium levels seem to prevent effective potassium therapy, so the test is especially important when a patient has a low serum potassium level but shows no positive response to administration of potassium.

Normal values: Serum magnesium levels range from 1.5 to 2.5 mEq per liter (2 mg per 100 ml). Values vary with different laboratory techniques.

Abnormal values: Lower than normal values are found with parathyroid, thyroid, and adrenal gland hyperactivity, and with malnutrition, chronic alcoholism, pancreatitis, and diuretic therapy. Higher than normal values are found with dehydration and with inactive adrenal glands.

MAKE-A-PICTURE STORY, see *Thematic Apperception*

MALABSORPTION, see *Xylose Tolerance*

MALARIA

Cases of malaria have increased in recent years as more and more people travel to areas of the world where the disease is endemic. There are four different types of parasites that cause the disease in humans: Plasmodium falciparum (the most serious), Plasmodium vivax, Plasmodium ovale, and Plasmodium malariae. The Anopheles mosquito is a carrier of the parasite, and its bite when infected spreads the disease. Blood is taken from a vein or fingertip and stained (with Wright's stain, Field's stain, or Giemsa's stain). The sample is then examined under the microscope for direct identification of malaria organisms.

When performed: When symptoms such as recurring fever, chills, anemia, and paroxysms suggest malaria; when a patient has recently returned from traveling in countries where the disease exists (such as West Africa).

Normal values: Normally there are no malaria organisms in the blood.

Abnormal values: Identification of any one of the various species of malaria parasites in a blood sample is indicative of infection.

MALE-FEMALE IDENTITY, see *Chromatin*

MALE SEX ORGAN FUNCTION, see *Testis Function*

MAMMOGRAPHY, see *Radiography*

MANGANESE

Recent research has indicated that people with epilepsy have lower than normal blood levels of the mineral manganese. It is not known whether decreased manganese in the blood is the cause of epilepsy or a result of the disease. Close relatives of patients with epilepsy also seem to have low blood manganese levels, although they may exhibit no symptoms of epilepsy. Because manganese is found in virtually all foods, it was once assumed that there could be no manganese deficiency. Adding extra manganese to the diet of a patient with epilepsy has, in a few cases, improved the patient's condition. Blood is taken from a vein and the whole blood is tested.

When performed: It may well become routine to test all patients with epilepsy for blood manganese levels.

Normal values: Normal manganese levels range from 15 to 50 mcg per liter.

Abnormal values: Patients with epilepsy, and their immediate relatives, average between 5 and 10 mcg per liter.

MAPLE SYRUP URINE DISEASE, see *Aminoaciduria*

MASTER TWO-STEP, see *Electrocardiogram*

MATERNITY, see *Disputed Parentage*; *Pregnancy*

MAXIMUM BREATHING CAPACITY, see *Pulmonary Function*

MAXIMUM EXPIRATORY FLOW RATE, see *Pulmonary Function*

MAXIMUM MIDEXPIRATORY FLOW RATE, see *Pulmonary Function*

MAXIMUM VOLUNTARY VENTILATION, see *Pulmonary Function*

MAZZINI, see *Syphilis*

MCH, see *Red Blood Cell Indices*

MCHC, see *Red Blood Cell Indices*

MCV, see *Red Blood Cell Indices*

MEAN CORPUSCULAR HEMOGLOBIN, see *Red Blood Cell Indices*

MEAN CORPUSCULAR HEMOGLOBIN CONCENTRATION, see *Red Blood Cell Indices*

MEAN CORPUSCULAR VOLUME, see *Red Blood Cell Indices*

MEASLES, see *Agglutination*

MELANA, see *Occult Blood*

MELANOGEN-MELANIN

Malignant melanoma is a skin condition of black spots that are believed to start from an inherited nevus (mole); it is the most dangerous of all skin cancers. Many patients with melanomas secrete colorless melanogen in the urine, which then turns to dark brown or black melanin after several hours' exposure to air. The addition of ferric chloride hastens the reaction. A single urine sample is used for testing.

When performed: When a patient has blue-black, brown-black or jet black moles or pigmentation on the skin, or when a light brown mole turns darker.

Normal values: No melanogen (turning to melanin) should be detected in urine.

Abnormal values: The presence of melanin in any quantity usually confirms the diagnosis of malignant melanoma. At times, a black-colored urine must be distinguished from alkaptonuria (see **Aminoaciduria**).

MELIOIDOSIS, see *Agglutination*

MENTAL DEPRESSION, see *Depression*

MENTAL STATUS, see *Cognitive Capacity Screening*

MERCURY

Mercury is a metallic element that can be toxic when taken into the body in sufficient amounts. Mercury can enter the body by inhalation if it is in the air; by contact with the skin (many skin ointments used to include mercury); by injection, as when it is used as a diuretic drug; and mostly by ingestion, as when eating fish containing even a trace of the metal. There are two different forms of mercury: the inorganic form (such as that used in thermometers), which causes vomiting, diarrhea, and kidney failure (most mercury is ultimately stored in the kidneys); and the organic form (such as that used in drugs), which causes weakness, brain damage, loss of balance, mental illness, and muscle pains.

When small amounts of mercury are taken into the body over long periods of time (years), no symptoms may appear until they build up to a toxic level. Urine is most frequently examined for mercury; blood from a vein may also be tested, as well as hair, nails, and other tissues.

When performed: On people who work with mercury (dental assistants, mirror makers, people who manufacture or use certain insecticides); with patients who seem to have mental illness, especially irritability or depression, when there is no known cause or provocation and when no psychiatric diagnosis can be made; when there is weakness, muscle tremors or cramps, brain damage, or kidney damage that cannot be diagnosed.

Normal values: There should be less than 10 mcg of mercury per 100 ml of urine and less than 2 mcg per 100 ml of blood. Hair and nails normally show a slight trace of the metal, usually less than 10 mcg per gram.

Abnormal values: While the amount of mercury varies tremendously in different individuals before it causes symptoms, in most instances a urine level greater than 20 mcg per 100 ml, a blood level greater than 20 mcg per 100 ml, or tissue amounts greater than 100 mcg per gram are indicative of mercury intoxication.

METANEPHRINS, see *Catecholamines*

METHANOL

Methanol (sometimes called methyl alcohol or wood alcohol) is sometimes ingested accidentally in place of ethanol (ethyl alcohol), the basis for liquors. One ounce of ethanol is usually metabolized and excreted by the body in three hours (depending on the quantity taken in). In contrast, it takes the body more than 24 hours to eliminate each ounce of methanol. More than an ounce of methanol can cause blindness and even death. Sterno is a solid form of methanol.

Isopropyl alcohol (regular rubbing alcohol) and ethylene glycol (the primary ingredient of automobile antifreeze) are also poisonous, but to a somewhat lesser degree than methanol. (Ethylene glycol causes oxalate crystals in the urine; see **Urinary Tract Calculus**.) Blood from a vein or urine may be tested.

When performed: When a patient has a combination of breathing and vision difficulties or is in a coma and no diagnosis can be made; when the ethyl **Alcohol** test is positive, but there are no signs of drunkenness.

Normal values: There should be no trace of methanol, isopropyl alcohol, or ethylene glycol in the blood or urine.

Abnormal values: Any amount found in the blood or urine is abnormal; values greater than 50 mg per 100 ml of blood can be fatal.

METHEMOGLOBIN, see *Hemoglobin*

METYRAPONE, see *Cortisol*

MICROBIAL CULTURE, see *Culture*

MIDDLE-EAR INFECTION, see *Tympanometry*

MILK ALLERGY, see *Agglutination*

MILK INTOLERANCE, see *Lactose Tolerance*

MINNESOTA MULTIPHASIC PERSONALITY INVENTORY (MMPI)

The MMPI is perhaps the most widely used test in clinical psychology; it is used to assess ostensibly normal subjects as well as those with alleged disabling personality traits. The test consists of 550 statements printed on separate cards (for example, "I wish I could be as happy as others seem to be," "I am sure I am being talked about," "Someone has been trying to influence my mind"). The subject sorts the cards into piles indicating whether he agrees, disagrees, or "cannot say."

Essentially, the test covers nine traditional psychiatric diagnostic categories: hypochondria, depression, hysteria, psychopathic deviate, masculine-feminine interest (homosexuality), paranoia, psychasthenia, schizophrenia, and hypomania. It has since been extended to cover many new diagnostic interpretations. The responses are assessed to provide a coded profile. For example, an affirmative answer to the statement "I think I would like the work of a librarian" is supposed to indicate feminine occupational identification. Certain statements are used to determine whether the subject is lying. For example, an affirmative response to the statement "My sex life is satisfactory" (a statement that is a component of the lie-scale section of the test) is considered an indication that all the patient's responses are questionable. One criticism of the original form of this test is that its standards are based on a sample of the city of Minneapolis rather than on a broader, more representative population. The test is particularly open to censure when it is used on individuals of diverse ethnic backgrounds.

When performed: The MMPI is used to uncover pathological tendencies as well as to reveal a profile of an individual's personality. It is also used for student counseling and screening of potential employees. Some clinics, usually those treating orthopedic problems such as bad back, perform the MMPI on all patients to help evaluate the psychological component of pain complaints.

Normal values: Similar patterns of responses in thousands of cases form the basis for coding individual profiles. The response profiles are used for differential diagnosis as well as for personality description.

Abnormal values: Certain response profiles are supposed to differentiate normal from pathological personalities (indicating paranoia, schizophrenia, depression, hypochondria, and other psychiatric conditions).

MIOSIS, see *Pupillary Reflex*

MITE INFESTATION, see *Scabies Infestation*

MMPI, see *Minnesota Multiphasic Personality Inventory*

MONONUCLEOSIS

The many and varied complaints of patients with infectious mononucleosis—including sore throat, headache, swollen glands (enlarged lymph nodes), abdominal pain, bleeding, and neurological problems—make diagnosis difficult. The disease was once thought to be spread by kissing and thus was called the "kissing disease." In infectious mononucleosis, the patient's antibody level reaction to sheep red blood cells rises. The heterophile antibody (an immunoglobulin) test is the primary aid for diagnosis. Blood is taken from a vein and the serum tested as in the **Agglutination** test. The Forssman antibody test is even more specific. There are several other "spot" tests to detect mononucleosis antibodies; most require only one drop of fingertip blood placed on a chemically treated spot on a slide (Mono-Diff, Mono-Test, Mono-Spot). A marked increase in atypical lymphocytes in a **Blood Cell Differential** also points to infectious mononucleosis.

When performed: When there is suspicion of infectious mononucleosis; to differentiate infectious mononucleosis from other diseases.

Normal values: Normally there may be very small amounts of antibody to sheep red blood cells (below a dilution of 1:112).

Abnormal values: Antibody levels are elevated to a dilution of 1:224 or more in approximately 70% of patients with mononucleosis; elevated levels may persist for weeks.

MOSENTHAL

The specific gravity of urine is usually a routine measurement; normally it should be high when the urine is concentrated (contains more solid matter), most frequently on awakening, and lower after a large amount of fluid is ingested. At times, however, more precise tests of specific gravity are required to pinpoint the location of a kidney problem; they are called urine concentration tests.

For the Mosenthal test, the patient cannot drink any liquids (the usual food diet is allowed) for 24 hours prior to testing. The first specimen of urine is voided on awakening and measured for specific gravity. The patient stays in bed for an additional hour and then voids again for another specific gravity measurement. The patient gets up and is active for one more hour, after which a third and final urine specimen is taken. Some doctors test only for specific gravity; others also perform a **Chloride** test on the urine.

The Fishberg test is a shortened version of the Mosenthal. Very little liquid is taken with dinner the night before the test and no food or liquids are taken during the night. When the patient awakens a urine sample is collected; two additional samples are taken an hour apart. The patient stays in bed the entire time. The test cannot be performed when a patient is taking diuretic drugs or certain hormones or is eating an unusual diet (especially one low in protein).

When performed: Whenever kidney disease is suspected; when adrenal or pituitary hormone problems, liver disease, or unexplainable edema (water retention) exists.

Normal values: No matter what version of the test is used, at least one urine sample should show a specific gravity of 1.025 or greater, indicating the kidney's ability to concentrate urine when liquids are withheld.

Abnormal values: A specific gravity value of less than 1.020 indicates kidney problems. As the specific gravity decreases in value, greater kidney pathology is indicated. On occasion, a low specific gravity will result from pituitary problems or the failure of the adrenals to produce antidiuretic hormone (ADH), but this can be distinguished from kidney disease by administering ADH to the patient and noting the response.

MOTOR DEVELOPMENT

There are several different measurements of infant motor development (how early in life and how well a child learns to use his muscles and coordinate his activities). The most popular is the Gesell Developmental Schedule, in which a child's physical activities are compared against a set of norms or standards determined by studying thousands of children during different stages of development. For example, at four weeks old, a child should be able to rotate his head and clench his fists. At five months, he should be able to grasp a rattle; at one year, he should be able to throw a ball; at four years, he should be able to walk up and down stairs properly and hop on one foot. There are "schedules" for ages up to six years.

Observations are also made of the child's language ability, drawing ability, and certain social activities such as personal grooming. The primary purpose of observation is to detect neurological (nervous system or muscle) pathology as early as possible. The Bayley Scale is another motor development measurement.

When performed: The Gesell test has become almost routine in pediatric examinations to aid in diagnosing developmental problems. It is also performed when a child appears to be slow in acquiring the usual developmental traits for his age (for example, not walking when expected to; not responding to stimuli).

Normal values: There are schedules (or expected standards) of physical activity for various ages, a few examples of which are described above (the schedules run into hundreds of observations).

Abnormal values: Failure to perform several activities expected at a given age; when a child appears to have multiple developmental problems, neurological or other pathology must be considered.

MUCIN CLOT, see *Synovial Fluid*

MULTIPLE MYELOMA, see *Bence-Jones Protein*

MUMPS, see *Agglutination*

MURAMIDASE, see *Lysozyme*

MUSCLE ENZYME, see *Aldolase*

MUSCLE REFLEX, see *Reflex*

MUSCLE STIMULATION, see *Electromyography*

MUSCLE TENSION, see *Electromyography*

MUSCULAR DYSTROPHY ENZYME, see *Creatine Phosphokinase*

MYASTHENIA GRAVIS, see *Tensilon*

MYCOSIS, see *Fungus*

MYELOGRAPHY (MYELOGRAM), see *Radiography*

MYELOMATOSIS, see *Bence-Jones Protein*

MYOGRAPHY, see *Electromyography*

MYOPIA, see *Visual Acuity*

NASAL AIRWAY RESISTANCE, see *Smell Function*

NEARSIGHTEDNESS, see *Visual Acuity*

NEONATAL HYPOTHYROID, see *Thyroid Function*

NEPHROCALCINOSIS, see *Urinary Tract Calculus*

NEPHROLITHIASIS, see *Urinary Tract Calculus*

NERVE CONDUCTION, see *Electromyography*

NERVOUS STRESS, see *Electromyography*

NIACIN (Vitamin B₃)

Skin rashes, headache, nervousness, diarrhea, loss of appetite, insomnia, and inflammation of the tongue are all symptoms of niacin (vitamin B₃) deficiency, Nicotinic acid and niacinamide are forms of this vitamin. Niacinamide is sometimes used in therapy because it causes fewer side effects. Niacin is found mostly in yeast, meats, fish, poultry, and eggs, and in small amounts in vegetables. Pellagra is the specific disease that may result from lack of sufficient niacin and is known in medicine as the 3-D disease: characterized by diarrhea, dermatitis, and dementia (mental depression). Niacin is measured by testing for its metabolic end products in the urine.

When performed: In mental illness, especially schizophrenia, mania, depression, and paranoia; when skin diseases cannot be easily diagnosed; in patients on vegetarian diets; with alcoholism.

Normal values: The metabolic end products of niacin should range from at least 0.6 to 1.59 mg in a 6-hour urine specimen.

Abnormal values: Less than 0.6 mg for a 6-hour urine specimen indicates a vitamin B$_3$ deficiency sufficient to cause disease (pellagra).

NICOTINIC ACID, see *Niacin*

NONMATERNITY, see *Disputed Parentage*

NONPATERNITY, see *Disputed Parentage*

NONPROTEIN NITROGEN (NPN), see *Urea Nitrogen*

NORADRENALIN, see *Catecholamines*

NOREPINEPHRINE, see *Catecholamines*

NPN, see *Urea Nitrogen*

NUCLEAR SCANNING

Nuclear scanning, or radionuclide organ imaging, may be performed on many parts of the body to aid in diagnosing and treating disease. Its primary function is to outline the size, shape, and exact location of an organ (liver, kidney, vein, etc.) or a chamber or duct within an organ. Nuclear scanning tests are also fairly precise in measuring organ function.

A radioactive material (radioisotope or radionuclide) is injected or ingested into the body; depending on the organ to be studied, it may be inserted into an arm vein or administered through a catheter (thin, hollow tube) that starts in an arm or leg vein or artery and is pushed through the blood vessels to the specific organ being tested. In a heart scan, for example, the catheter may start in the arm or the neck and end directly inside the heart chamber being studied. To test the thyroid, a patient drinks radioactive iodine. Various chemicals are known to select certain body organs and after being made radioactive they can be detected within the organ by rectilinear scanners or gamma cameras, both of which work on the same principle as the Geiger counter in detecting uranium. A faster modification of the process is called scintography.

The amount of radioactivity in the injected chemicals is so small as to cause no known harmful effects to the body. Virtually all radioactivity is gone within a day or so. The scanning machines that detect the radioactivity do not give off any radiation.

In many instances, the radioactivity is visualized on a photographic plate or an X-ray plate. Sometimes a computer printout is made on paper outlining the organ being studied. The results show the size and shape of the organ as well as any part of the organ that failed to pick up radioactive material—usually indicating a defect (disease, tumor). Any excess of radioactivity in an area usually means the organ is enlarged or hyperactive. Through measurement of the flow of radioactive material through an organ, the function of that organ can be determined. When the kidneys are tested, measurement of blood flowing into and out of the kidney is called a renogram; measurement of the size, shape, and position of the kidney is called a renal scan. Usually both kidneys are measured at the same time to better detect which kidney, if only one, is affected.

Most often the nuclear scanning test is referred to by the organ being studied; examples are discussed below.

Brain scan: Radioactive chemicals (mostly technetium) are used for brain imaging; normal brain tissue will not pick up most of the tracer material. A concentration of radioactive material usually indicates an increased number of blood vessels and a disease process. The scanning is performed twice, immediately after the injection of radioactive material and then 24 hours later.

Bone scan: Usually radioactive strontium is used (since it replaces calcium) and a uniform uptake (or concentration) throughout all the bones is normal. An increased concentration in a specific area is abnormal and usually represents cancer, but arthritis and fractures can sometimes give a similar picture. Radioactive gallium is used in testing for hidden bone infections, since gallium seems to seek out inflammatory tissue. Usually a bone scan is performed a few hours after injection of the material.

Lung scan: There are two kinds of lung scanning: a perfusion scan and a ventilation scan. They may be performed separately or together to aid in diagnosis. The perfusion scan is more common. Radioactive albumin is injected into a vein and the scanning is performed immediately. The primary purpose of a perfusion scan is to diagnose pulmonary embolism. When the two different lung scans are performed together, it is also possible to evaluate pulmonary function in emphysema and other lung obstructions, to locate a growth and follow the course of that growth before and after treatment, to measure the size of the heart, and to discern areas of infection and lung collapse. The ventilation scan is performed by having the patient breathe in radioactive xenon gas and then passing the scanner over the lungs. Inhaled radioactive xenon can show normal or abnormal bronchial passageways and areas of the lung that do not receive air.

Liver scan: Nuclear scanning is probably the best way to study the liver without surgery. Radioactive gold or rose bengal (a dye) is injected into a vein. Normally the chemical is absorbed by the liver within 20 minutes and shows a uniform appearance when viewed by the scanner. If, however, there is pathology (growth, cirrhosis, or abscess), that area will not take up the chemical and the absence of radioactivity indicates disease.

Spleen scan: The same chemicals used for a liver scan are often used to visualize the spleen; however, radioactive red blood cells (erythrocytes) give an even better image (since the spleen's function is to remove ineffective erythrocytes from the blood). The test is used to help diagnose an unknown mass in the upper left portion of the abdomen, to evaluate the size and functioning of the spleen, and to diagnose spleen injury. Spleen scanning takes place about four hours after red blood cell injection.

Pancreas scan: A radioactive selenium-amino acid compound is injected in a vein. The pancreas normally takes up this amino acid immediately and the radioactive element allows imaging of the organ in about ten minutes. Pancreatic disease is difficult to diagnose, and this test helps detect cancer, cysts, and infection by the organ's failure to show absorption of the radioactive material.

Heart or cardiac scan: Radioactive thallium is injected into a vein and is absorbed by heart tissue, allowing visualization of the size and shape of the heart. This test is particularly valuable when pericarditis (excessive fluid around the heart) is suspected. Scanning takes place immediately after injection of the chemical. Other radioactive chemicals are used to outline the inside chambers of the heart. A blood pool scan shows heart contractions clearly and can help indicate the amount of damage after a heart attack.

Vein scan: Various radioactive chemicals injected into a vein will be absorbed in blood clots if a thrombus or phlebitis is present. The clot is easily visualized. The test may also predict patients who are prone to thromboembolism.

Thyroid scan: See **Thyroid Function**.

Spinal fluid scan: Radioactive albumin is injected into the lower-back spinal fluid space (see **Cerebrospinal Fluid**) and observed as it passes around the cord into the brain spaces. The chemical takes about 24 hours to reach the brain area and remains there for two to three days. This test is especially valuable in diagnosing hydrocephalus (abnormally large head); it is also indicated when there is suspicion of a spinal fluid leak. The test is sometimes called cisternography, spinal cord scan, or intrathecal scan.

Placental scan: When there is doubt about the exact position of the fetus during pregnancy, the injection of an extremely tiny dose of radioactive albumin will help show the location of the placenta so as to place the fetus. When there is suspicion of intrauterine bleeding, usually due to a damaged placenta, this test will help diagnose the condition and can be life-saving to the patient.

In some cases, instead of a diagram or illustration of the radioactivity, a counter is placed over the organ and the amount of radioactivity is "counted" and recorded as to its intensity. This technique is often used in testing organ function, since it is easier and continuous.

When performed: In general, scanning is performed when it is necessary to visualize an organ and to follow the progress of certain diseases. More specific indications for nuclear scanning are noted in the descriptions of the scanning procedures above.

Normal values: Normal values are noted in the specific scanning descriptions above.

Abnormal values: Whether an organ should or should not pick up and reflect radioactivity is discussed under each organ-scanning procedure. The normality, abnormality, and degree of abnormality are determined by a physician with extensive experience in the field.

Note: Radioimmunoassay is a technique (not a specific test) which uses radionuclides (as used in scanning) for measuring minute quantities of hormones, certain drugs, and antigens that can cause disease (see **Agglutination; RAST**). It is another method to verify hormone deficiency or excess, drug toxicity, allergy, and infections.

O₂, see *Oxygen*

OCCULT BLOOD

In medicine the word "occult" means present but invisible. Thus occult blood procedures test for blood that can be seen only through microscopic or chemical examination. Virtually all body fluids, excretions, and secretions can be tested for occult blood; most often the test is performed on feces and urine. It has been proposed that if everyone's feces were properly tested for occult blood twice a year, almost all bowel cancer could be eliminated.

A person can lose about an ounce of blood a day from the bowel (amounting to a pint in two weeks) without noticing any bleeding. In contrast, visible bleeding occurs when more than 2 ounces of blood enter the bowel (from a bleeding ulcer, from a growth in the colon or large intestine, or from hemorrhoids). When that blood mixes with the stomach acid in the bowel, it turns black and is termed melena. Thus a general assumption is that black, tarry bowel movements indicate bleeding somewhere in the upper intestinal tract, while bright red blood indicates lower-bowel and rectal bleeding.

There are three different tests for occult blood: guaiac (Hemoccult), orthotoluidine, and benzidine. The orthotoluidine test is the most sensitive but will give a false positive result when the patient's diet includes meat. The guaiac test does not react to dietary meat but is the least sensitive. In most instances, a patient is told not to eat any meat or even to brush his teeth for at least three days before the test, since the slightest trace of blood from meat or from irritation of the gums can give a false positive test.

When performed: Whenever gastrointestinal or kidney disease is suspected; whenever a patient has an anemia that cannot be diagnosed.

Normal values: Urine, feces, and other body secretions should show no occult blood.

Abnormal values: A positive occult blood test, after eliminating all extraneous causes (brushing the teeth, irritating the throat, blowing the nose too hard, meat diet, taking excessive amount of iron pills), is considered abnormal. Occult blood can be found in the bowel with patients taking aspirin or other drugs that irritate the stomach. Alcoholic gastritis may also cause a positive test. Eating beets will color the feces red but will not cause a positive test. A positive urine occult blood test usually indicates pathology somewhere in the urinary tract, from the kidneys to the bladder to the ducts that carry the urine.

OCULAR HYPERTENSION, see *Tonometry*

OCULAR MUSCLE, see *Strabismus*

OLFACTORY PERCEPTION, see *Smell Function*

OPHTHALMOSCOPY, see *Fundoscopy*

ORGANIC PHOSPHATE POISONING, see *Cholinesterase*

ORGAN IMAGING, see *Computerized Tomography*; *Nuclear Scanning*; *Ultrasound*

ORGAN TRANSPLANT, see *HL-A Antigen*

ORTHOTOLUIDINE, see *Occult Blood*

OSMOLALITY

Osmolality is a measure of the osmotic pressure of a liquid. In medicine osmotic pressure indicates the amount of dissolved material (minerals, hormones, etc.) in a body fluid, most commonly blood or urine. Large amounts of sodium, sugars, fats, and other substances increase the blood's osmolality; in fact, the amount of sodium alone in the blood can sometimes be used as a reasonable measure of serum osmolality. Blood osmolality regulates body water (the feeling of thirst, when water is needed, and the control of urine output), and it depends primarily on blood electrolytes (see **Chloride**; **Potassium**; **Sodium**). Blood is taken from a vein and the serum is tested. Urine is also tested for osmolality.

The osmolality test is considered more accurate than the urine specific gravity test (see **Mosenthal**), which offers somewhat similar measurements (specific gravity measures the size of the particles). A common method of testing for osmolality is to measure the exact degree at which the liquid freezes, since soluble particles in a liquid affect the freezing point.

When performed: When dehydration is suspected; in alcoholism; when excessive amounts of fats are in the blood (hyperlipidemia); in uncontrolled diabetes and in unexplained instances of edema (water retention); to measure the effects of intravenous therapy.

Normal values: Normally osmolality should range from 280 to 295 mOsm per liter (about the same as normal plasma) in blood and 300 to 1,200 mOsm per liter of urine.

Abnormal values: Levels are increased (hyperosmolality) with water loss (vomiting, diarrhea, excess sweating) or inadequate water intake (300 mOsm per liter is considered moderate to severe dehydration), with brain or kidney damage, and with diabetes insipidus. Decreased levels occur when excess water is taken in or administered (such as with intravenous therapy) and when diuretic drugs are used (which cause excretion of a great deal of sodium ions, lessening the amount of blood electrolytes). Markedly decreased levels in the urine indicate failure of the kidney's concentrating ability.

OTIS, see *Intelligence Quotient*

OVA AND PARASITE, see *Feces Examination*

OVULATION, see *Body Temperature*

OVULATION TIME, see *Tackmeter*

OXALATE

Eating many foods that naturally contain the chemical oxalate (sorrel, spinach, cabbage, tomatoes, rhubarb, and even chocolate) usually has no adverse effect; in some people, however, it can cause hyperoxaluria (an abnormally excessive amount of oxalate in the urine). If it then combines with calcium, oxalate can on occasion cause kidney stones. A rare inherited condition known as primary hyperoxaluria or oxalosis (as distinguished from secondary or ordinary hyperoxaluria) causes kidney infections and high blood pressure. Oxalate is measured in urine. Since oxalate levels can be lowered by altering the diet, the test aids not only in diagnosis but also in following the progress of treatment.

When performed: The test is used whenever a patient has symptoms of kidney or bladder stones. It is also performed when there are certain intestinal inflammation problems that do not respond to therapy, when the intestine has been operated on for cancer or ulcers, or when, in rare instances, an intestinal bypass procedure is performed to promote weight loss. (It is believed that the presence of excessive oxalates after surgery represents a vitamin B_6 deficiency from poor intestinal absorption.) Oxalate levels are measured when there is suspicion of ethylene glycol (automobile antifreeze) or oxalic acid (bleach) poisoning.

Normal values: Oxalate levels normally range from 0 to 40 mg per 24-hour specimen of urine.

Abnormal values: Levels greater than 50 mg per 24-hour sample of urine are considered abnormal. With hyperoxaluria, the urine usually shows white, cloudy formations.

OXYGEN

Oxygen in the blood is measured in a variety of ways. The *oxygen content* is the amount of the gas actually present in the blood. The *oxygen capacity* is the amount of oxygen that would be found in the blood if all it could hold were present. Both measures indicate just how much oxygen is available to support life, or the percentage of oxygen saturation of the blood. Most often blood oxygen is measured as the *partial pressure of oxygen* (Po_2), sometimes called *oxygen tension*.

Oxygen is rarely tested alone; it is almost always measured along with the blood's **Carbon Dioxide** (CO_2) and **pH** (hydrogen ions that indicate how acid the blood is). Once the Po_2 and the pH are known, the amount of oxygen attached to hemoglobin (hemoglobin saturation) can be determined. These three different tests are known as the blood gas group.

Whole blood is taken from an artery for most oxygen testing; in an emergency it can be taken from a vein to measure content or saturation. The sample must be collected in a syringe that is coated inside with oil to prevent any air from reaching the blood; the needle tip must be sealed immediately and the syringe packed in ice. (A new device claims to measure Po_2 simply by touching the skin.) Elderly patients should be reclining when the blood is taken, since blood oxygen is lowest in that position and yields a truer value.

When performed: Primarily in respiratory diseases and in conditions that affect the lungs and interfere with transfer of oxygen to the blood; to determine if oxygen therapy will be effective; when there is heart failure; when there is suspected hypnotic or narcotic drug overdose; as a means of better evaluating kidney problems.

Normal values: Normal values for the different measures of oxygen are as follows:

Oxygen tension (Po_2): 85 to 105 mm Hg (after 40 years of age it may be lower.)

Oxygen content: 15 to 23 volumes % for arterial blood and 10 to 16 volumes % for venous blood.

Oxygen capacity: 16 to 24 volumes % (levels depend on how much hemoglobin is present, since each gram of hemoglobin holds 1.39 ml of oxygen).

Oxygen saturation: from 94% to 100% of capacity for arterial blood and from 60% to 85% of capacity for venous blood.

Abnormal values: Oxygen values are decreased (hypoxemia) with any chronic obstructive lung disease (such as emphysema) or during an asthmatic attack. Almost any respiratory complication of disease can reduce oxygen utilization as reflected by lowered oxygen values for all the tests. Polycythemia (too many red blood cells) will also lower oxygen values. Exercise can decrease the amount of oxygen in the blood.

PACKED BLOOD CELL VOLUME, see *Hematocrit*

PAH CLEARANCE (SODIUM P-AMINOHIPPURIC), see *Creatinine*

PANCREAS ENZYME, see *Amylase*

PANCREAS SCAN, see *Nuclear Scanning*

PAPANICOLAOU (PAP), see *Cytology*

PARACENTESIS, see *Thoracentesis*

PARASITE, see *Feces Examination*

PARATHYROID, see *Calcium*

PARENTHOOD EXCLUSION, see *Disputed Parentage*

PAROXYSMAL NOCTURNAL HEMOGLOBINURIA, see *HAM*

PARTIAL PRESSURE OF CARBON DIOXIDE, see *Carbon Dioxide*

PARTIAL PRESSURE OF OXYGEN, see *Oxygen*

PARTIAL THROMBOPLASTIN TIME (PTT)

Thromboplastin is one of the 12 factors in the body that cause blood to clot. The partial thromboplastin time (PTT) test measures the efficacy of eight of those factors, primarily Factors VIII and IX (the antihemophilia factors). It is gradually replacing the older **Bleeding and Clotting Time** tests. Blood is drawn from a vein and plasma is examined. The test serves the same function as the blood clotting time which must be measured immediately after the blood is taken; the advantage of the PTT is that the blood sample may be measured later in a laboratory.

When performed: In diagnosing hemophilia; to monitor therapy of hemophilia; when heparin is prescribed.

Normal values: Normal partial thromboplastin time averages 35 to 50 seconds, depending on the laboratory.

Abnormal values: Elevated PTT levels (more than 50 seconds) occur with hemophilia and with patients taking heparin.

PATCH, see *Skin Reaction*

PATERNITY, see *Disputed Parentage*

PBI, see *Thyroid Function*

PCG, see *Phonocardiogram*

PCO₂, see *Carbon Dioxide*

PETT, see *Computerized Tomography*

PEG, see *Radiography*

PELLAGRA, see *Niacin*

PENILE PLETHYSMOGRAPHY, see *Plethysmography*

PEP, see *Systolic Time Intervals*

PERFUSION SCAN, see *Nuclear Scanning*

PERIMETRY, see *Visual Field*

PERIPHERAL VISION, see *Visual Field*

PERITONEOSCOPY, see *Endoscopy*

PERSONALITY, see *Depression*; *Minnesota Multiphasic Personality Inventory*; *Rorschach*; *Thematic Apperception*

PERTHES, see *Tourniquet Test for Varicose Veins*

PETECHIAE, see *Capillary Fragility*

pH

pH is a measure of how much hydrogen gas is in the blood; it reflects the number of hydrogen ions that are present per liter. A pH of 7, which is neutral (neither acid nor alkaline), means there are 100 nanoequivalents of hydrogen ions per liter of blood. The body functions best when the blood pH is 7.40—that is, when it contains about 40 nanoequivalents of hydrogen ions per liter. Therefore, the blood is normally very slightly alkaline (on the base side when considered on an acid-base relationship).

The balance is so delicate that when the pH goes below 7.38 (a difference of only 2 nanoequivalents of hydrogen: far less than a billionth of a gram), normal body functions are disrupted and the pathological condition of acidemia (acidosis) exists. The body immediately struggles to correct the condition, which can be fatal if allowed to persist. A drop in pH also causes severe constriction of arteries and a lack of oxygen to tissues. Should hydrogen ions be lost from the body (or neutralized) and the blood pH rise above 7.44, the opposite pathology occurs—a condition known as alkalemia (alkalosis). If the alteration is caused primarily by bicarbonate, it is called metabolic; if the change is caused by carbon dioxide, it is called respiratory. Either condition reflects an acid-base balance disturbance.

Since most normal metabolic reactions in the body tend to create acids, the blood is always slightly alkaline (to neutralize the acids). Breathing out carbon dioxide (which is acid) also helps keep the pH properly balanced. Preferably, blood from an artery is tested; properly collected venous blood can be measured in emergency situations. The blood must not be exposed to air. The pH is also measured in urine, spinal fluid, lung fluid, semen, and many other body secretions.

When performed: Almost always in conjunction with **Carbon Dioxide** and **Bicarbonate** tests and frequently with **Oxygen** testing; whenever there are respiratory or kidney problems that cannot be positively diagnosed; when a patient is in a coma or very confused; following vomiting or diarrhea; with severe muscle cramps; when certain drug poisoning is suspected.

Normal values: Normal pH in the blood ranges from 7.38 to 7.44. The body will not survive a pH lower than 6.8 or higher than 7.8.

Abnormal values: Levels below 7.35 indicate acidosis: either respiratory (from a lung condition that prevents the normal exchange of oxygen and carbon dioxide from the blood to the air, such as asthma, emphysema, an injury that causes a blood clot in the lung, or fractured ribs) or metabolic (from drug poisoning such as aspirin or from diabetes, diarrhea, or kidney disease). A pH above 7.45 indicates alkalosis: either respiratory (from deliberate fast breathing, certain drugs, or liver disease) or metabolic (from taking diuretics, steroids, or alkaline antacids for ulcers or burning stomach, or from vomiting or adrenal disease).

Urine pH is normally acid, especially on arising, but it becomes more acid (sometimes abnormally so) with kidney disease or lung disease, and after taking certain drugs or eating a great deal of meat. Urine becomes less acid (and sometimes alkaline) with various drugs and when the diet is high in vegetables and fruits. Spinal fluid is normally alkaline but becomes acid when excessive drugs are administered and in certain lung diseases. Most other body fluids are alkaline; when they become acid, pathology is usually indicated (an acid semen means decreased fertility).

PHENOLSULFONPHTHALEIN (PSP)

Kidney function is often tested by injecting phenolsulfonphthalein (PSP) dye into the bloodstream and measuring the amount of the dye excreted in the urine after specific time intervals (15 minutes, 30 minutes, one hour, and two hours). The test does not depend on the amount of urine produced. Six milligrams (1 ml) of the dye is injected intravenously half an hour after the patient has drunk two glasses of water.

When performed: The test is used whenever kidney disease or urinary tract obstruction is suspected and with edema (water retention) or hypertension. It may also be performed with catheters inserted in each ureter (the tube that carries urine from each kidney to the bladder) to discover if only one kidney is damaged.

Normal values: Normally about 25% of the dye is excreted in the urine in the first 15 minutes, 50% in the first 30 minutes, 65% after the first hour, and 75% by the second hour.

Abnormal values: Excretion of PSP may be reduced in kidney disease and urinary tract obstruction. Excretion of PSP may be increased in liver disease and high blood pressure. Many drugs (diuretics, aspirin, penicillin, certain vitamins) can cause abnormal PSP results.

PHENOTYPING, see *Lipoproteins*

PHENYLALANINE, see *Phenylketonuria*

PHENYLKETONURIA (PKU)

Phenylketonuria (PKU) is an inherited amino acid enzyme deficiency that can cause mental retardation because of the body's inability to metabolize a protein amino acid, phenylalanine, which is then abnormally found in the urine. It occurs once in every 10,000 births and is most common among people from northern Ireland and western Scotland. Early treatment of this metabolic disorder—by a diet low in phenylalanine (using synthetic proteins in place of plant and animal proteins)—can prevent mental retardation; thus the testing of newborn infants is essential to early diagnosis and treatment. A very small amount of phenylalanine is necessary for normal growth, and children differ markedly in how much they can eat without showing symptoms.

The primary test for phenylketonuria is the blood Guthrie Bacterial Inhibition Assay (GBIA). A small amount of blood is usually drawn from the infant's heel for testing. The test cannot be performed until at least 24 hours after the infant has had its first milk meal. (Breast-fed infants must be tested again after one month.) Urine can also be tested for PKU, but blood will show a positive reaction much sooner than urine. If the Guthrie test is positive, a blood phenylalanine analysis is performed to confirm the diagnosis.

The dinitrophenylhydrazine (DNPH) test and ferric chloride urine test help detect PKU as well as other inherited metabolic defects. There are also special plastic strips coated with chemicals that turn color when dipped into the urine (or even placed on a wet diaper) of a child with phenylketonuria, but occasionally they give a false positive reaction.

When performed: Testing of newborn infants for PKU has become mandatory in most states. The test is also used when mental retardation seems evident.

Normal values: Normally there are less than 4 mg per 100 ml of demonstrable phenylalanine in the blood.

Abnormal values: When a child has PKU, the blood concentration of phenylalanine is kept between 3 and 7 mg per 100 ml. A concentration greater than 20 mg per 100 ml indicates a metabolic disorder. The urine will show 100 mcg per ml or more with PKU.

PHEOCHROMOCYTOMA, see *Catecholamines*

PHLEBOGRAPHY, see *Radiography*

PHLEBORHEOGRAPHY, see *Plethysmography*

PHLEGM, see *Sputum*

PHONOCARDIOGRAM (PCG)

The phonocardiogram (PCG) is similar to the **Apexcardiogram** (ACG), in that it uses a measuring apparatus called a transducer, which records on paper a representation of the heart sounds—especially those made by the heart valves when closing. The major difference between the PCG and the ACG is the graphic tracing of the heart sounds. The PCG is illustrated by a continuous series of short wavy lines (which actually look like vibrations); the stronger the sound, the greater and larger the line vibration recording from the base line. The ACG is illustrated by a continuous rising and falling line (more like a series of large waves). The PCG is always recorded along with an ACG and a standard **Electrocardiogram** (ECG) in order to identify the exact position of the heart (contraction, relaxation) at the time of the sound.

When performed: When abnormal heart sounds need to be recorded for permanent records; to confirm or differentiate the sounds heard through the stethoscope; after surgical replacement of heart valves to determine success and performance.

Normal values: The PCG (especially in conjunction with the ECG) shows a standard vibration pattern for heart sounds when the heart valves are normal in size and length.

Abnormal values: Heart valve disease (aortic stenosis, mitral stenosis, etc.) shows a unique change from the normal pattern. There is also a specific pattern when the heart is enlarged—to the point where the two normal heart sounds are recorded as one.

PHOSPHATASE, see *Acid Phosphatase*; *Alkaline Phosphatase*

PHOSPHATES, see *Phosphorus*

PHOSPHOLIPIDS, see *Lipids*

PHOSPHORUS

Phosphorus metabolism is directly related to calcium metabolism and is associated with many body functions, most controlled by the parathyroid glands. Ninety percent of the phosphorus in the body is stored in the skeleton. Approximately 1 g of phosphorus is ingested daily by the average adult; primarily from dairy foods, meat, nuts and vegetables. Although the test is reported as phosphorus, usually phosphate ions (phosphorus combined with something else such as oxygen phosphates) are measured. Blood is collected from an arm vein and the serum is examined. Phosphorus is also tested in urine and feces.

When performed: In kidney disease, hypoparathyroidism, suspected vitamin D deficiency (rickets), and undiagnosed nerve and muscle disease.

Normal values: Normal phosphorus levels range from 2.5 to 4.5 mg per 100 ml of serum (higher in children).

Abnormal values: Phosphorus levels may be increased in kidney disease, hypoparathyroidism, conditions of bone destruction and repair (healing fractures, certain bone diseases), and hypervitaminosis D (excess vitamin D), and sometimes in patients taking Dilantin, pituitrin, or heparin. Phosphorus levels may be decreased in certain rare diseases of the kidney tubules, alcoholism, hyperparathyroidism, and vitamin deficiency. Increased urine and feces phosphorus usually reflects a decrease in the serum.

PHOTOMOTOGRAPHY, see *Thyroid Function*

PHYTOHEMAGGLUTININ

Phytohemagglutinins are unique plant products that can cause changes in blood cells. The phytohemagglutinin test can help discover carriers of cystic fibrosis (of the pancreas), a generalized inherited disease that affects the **Sweat** glands and the lungs. It is believed that one out of 20 people carry the gene that induces the disease. The disease can now be controlled most of the time with antibiotics. Blood from a vein is taken and certain white blood cells are tested.

When performed: When cystic fibrosis (sometimes called mucoviscidosis) is suspected; whenever there is a persistent chest infection, especially lung congestion, in childhood or adolescence; when a patient has excessive sweating problems or malabsorption problems.

Normal values: Lymphocytes (white blood cells) exposed to phytohemagglutinin show a marked increase in the amount of proteins they contain.

Abnormal values: Patients with cystic fibrosis show a marked decrease in the amount of proteins in lymphocyte cells; carriers of cystic fibrosis show a small decrease, as opposed to the normally expected large increase.

PINHOLE, see *Visual Acuity*

PIN PRICK, see *Sensory*

PITUITARY GONADOTROPIN, see *Testis Function*

PKU, see *Phenylketonuria*

PLACENTAL LACTOGEN

Human placental lactogen (HPL), also known as human chorionic somatomammotrophin (HCS), is a hormone produced by the placenta (the blood supply around the fetus during pregnancy). It first appears in the blood after about the fifth week of pregnancy and gradually increases in amount until the baby is born, after which it disappears. Its appearance and gradual increase are an indication of normal pregnancy. Blood is taken from a vein and the serum is tested.

When performed: The HPL test is used whenever there is suspicion of trouble during pregnancy, especially if the patient has a sudden onset of vaginal bleeding. It has been suggested that the test be routinely performed during all pregnancies as a means of detecting potential miscarriage.

Normal values: No HPL is usually found until after the fifth week of pregnancy. At that time about 0.5 mcg per ml can be detected. The level then rises to between 7 and 10 mcg per ml just before delivery.

Abnormal values: Slightly increased values may be found with a large placenta (multiple births), but the test is not a positive indicator. A sudden decrease in HPL during pregnancy is considered a warning sign that a miscarriage is about to occur, usually because the fetus either is abnormal or is having some difficulty (such as insufficient oxygen or separation of the placenta from the uterus). Certain rare tumors may cause an increased amount of HPL in the blood.

PLACENTAL SCAN, see *Nuclear Scanning*; *Ultrasound*

PLASMA PROTEINS, see *Albumin/Globulin*

PLASMA RENIN ACTIVITY, see *Renin*

PLATELET COUNT

Platelets, or thrombocytes, are minuscule bodies (less than half the size of red blood cells) that are essential to the blood-clotting process. They are manufactured in bone marrow at the rate of about 100,000 each day. When bleeding occurs, platelets group or clump together (aggregate), swell up, stick to the injured area, and attempt to act as plugs to stop the bleeding. The normal life span of platelets is about eight days. Only one drop of blood is necessary for examination and may be taken from the fingertip, heel, or earlobe or from a tube of blood drawn for other tests. Platelets are usually counted manually under the microscope; electronic counting is also performed. Platelets are also examined for size (young, larger platelets are more effective for clotting).

When performed: When there are obvious bleeding tendencies; before surgical procedures or tooth extractions; with fractures; to check liver function; when polycythemia or certain kinds of anemia are suspected.

Normal values: There should be between 150,000 and 500,000 platelets per cu mm (lower for children). Normal values vary with different laboratory methods.

Abnormal values: Platelets are usually increased (more than 500,000 per cu mm) in rheumatoid arthritis, most cancers, trauma (hemorrhage), polycythemia, and some anemias (iron deficiency). They are decreased in bleeding tendencies (usually less than 20,000 per cu mm before bleeding occurs), purpura (a condition in which even the slightest bruise causes a black-and-blue mark from bleeding under the skin), some anemias, certain leukemias, and infectious mononucleosis.

Note: The newly developed platelet aggregation test (Aggregometer) helps distinguish between inherited (hemophilia, Von Willebrand's disease) and acquired bleeding problems. Drugs such as aspirin and aspirin-like products used for arthritis and generalized pain can keep platelets from aggregating and thus cause bleeding. This new test is also used as an indication of susceptibility to stroke in older people.

PLETHYSMOGRAPHY

Venous thrombosis (a clot attached to the wall of a vein), usually in a deep vein of the leg (and far more common in the left leg than in the right, for reasons as yet unknown), is becoming a common illness. Deep-vein thrombosis (and its potential consequence, pulmonary embolism or lung clot) frequently follows surgical procedures when patients must lie quietly for long periods after the operation. Phlebography (see **Radiography**) is the best way to diagnose deep-vein thrombosis (thrombophlebitis); however, when X-ray is difficult or when it is impossible to locate a vein in the foot for injection of a radio-opaque dye (because of excessive swelling, low pain threshold, etc.), venous impedence plethysmography is used. This is a noninvasive technique (the skin is not broken with injections) and is a safe, fairly reliable way to test for thrombosis.

In venous impedence plethysmography, a standard blood pressure cuff with measuring wires is connected to an impedence analyzer, which records the blood flow through the vein around the area of the leg where the clot is suspected. The blood pressure cuff is inflated to create pressure around the upper leg and thus slow or stop the flow of blood in the veins below the cuff. The pressure is released suddenly and the rate of venous blood flow is recorded. The test can be performed at home, in a doctor's office, or at the bedside of a hospitalized patient.

Penile plethysmography, using similar equipment, is used to differentiate psychological from physical **Impotence.**

When performed: Whenever there is swelling of the leg (usually but not always painful) that cannot be specifically diagnosed; prior to and following extensive surgical procedures, especially when the patient has been forced to lie on the operating table for a long period of time; whenever patients are bed-ridden for more than several days at a time; as a screening test for the prevention of thrombosis and pulmonary embolism and occasionally to follow the progress of the treatment of a clot; in cases of impotence.

Normal values: After the pressure in the blood pressure cuff is applied, the impedence analyzer should show a slow steady rise as the lower veins fill up but are unable to empty; as soon as the pressure is released, a sudden surge of blood into all the leg veins should be recorded.

Abnormal values: When a thrombus (clot) is present a vein will show very slow filling, and when the pressure above the vein is released the sudden surge of blood will not be recorded.

PLEURAL FLUID, see *Thoracentesis*

PLUMBISM, see *Lead*

PNEUMOENCEPHALOGRAPHY, see *Radiography*

PNEUMONIA, see *Complement Fixation*

PNEUMOTACHOMETER, see *Smell Function*

POLIOMYELITIS, see *Complement Fixation*

PORPHYRINS

Porphyrins are pigments that come from red blood cells and from the liver; when present in the urine they indicate disease (porphyria). Erythropoietic (red blood cell) porphyria is a rare, inherited condition characterized by the excretion of red-tinted urine shortly after birth. Hepatic (liver) porphyria may be inherited or acquired after birth as a consequence of drug use, alcoholism, or exposure to certain chemicals such as lead and fungicides. Virtually all people who have excessive porphyrins in their system are hypersensitive to sunlight. Exposure to sun results in edema, blisters, and other skin lesions, mostly ulcers and scarring. Other symptoms that occur with porphyria include generalized body pains (most commonly in the stomach), confusion, and convulsions. During an acute attack, a patient may have high blood pressure, an extremely rapid pulse, and fever.

The porphyrin test measures a number of different types of porphyrins (such as coproporphyrins, protoporphyrins, and uroporphyrins); it is usually not necessary to distinguish the type of porphyrin to establish a diagnosis. Two specific products that immediately precede the formation of porphyrins are porphobilinogen and delta aminolevulinic acid, called ALA (see **Lead**). Determination of these specific products helps pinpoint the diagnosis by showing whether the porphyria is erythropoietic or hepatic, inherited or acquired. A 24-hour sample of urine is the most common test. Porphyrins may also be measured in the feces, in the blood serum taken from a vein, and in red blood cells alone.

When performed: Primarily when a patient complains of reddish or reddish purple urine; when there is photosensitivity, hyperpigmentation, ulceration of the skin, excessive hair growth, undiagnosable stomach pains, unexplained convulsions, and other nervous disease manifestations that cannot be otherwise diagnosed; as an indication of a possible acute attack of porphyria and as a measure of progress while treating the disease; as an aid in testing for lead poisoning.

Normal values: Normally there are no porphyrins in the urine and no more than 1,000 mcg in a 24-hour feces specimen. There may be up to 100 mcg per 100 ml in red blood cells and up to 60 mcg per 100 ml of blood serum.

Abnormal values: Porphyrins are increased in the urine in porphyria, liver disease, certain cancers, and lead poisoning. They may also be increased with psychic trauma, menstruation, and pregnancy. Eating beets or blackberries or taking certain laxatives containing phenolsulfonphthalein (Ex-Lax), danthron, or cascara may give a false porphyrin-like color to the urine, as will certain azo-dye urinary anesthetics (Pyridium) and rifampin, an antibiotic. Patients who are malingering have been known to add ketchup or tomato juice to their urine in order to simulate illness.

POSITRON EMISSION TRANSAXIAL TOMOGRAPHY, see *Computerized Tomography*

POTASSIUM

Potassium is a blood electrolyte (see **Sodium**) that is essential to maintaining the proper balance of fluids within body cells. (Sodium acts in the same manner but is responsible for the water *surrounding* the body cells.) Potassium is particularly important to help carry out enzyme reactions throughout the body and to regulate heart muscle action. The typical daily diet contains about 3 g of potassium (less than half as much as sodium), but the body excretes almost all of it. Foods richest in potassium include dates, apricots, bananas, oranges, and tomatoes. Most problems come from too little potassium in the body, a condition caused more by reactions to drugs than by disease or lack of the mineral in the diet. Very little potassium is lost in sweat (which contains large amounts of sodium).

Blood is taken from a vein and the serum is examined. In this test particularly, but also in many others, the common practice of asking the patient to clench and open the fist (to help find a vein in the arm) or leaving the tourniquet on too long can cause great errors in measurement. Potassium is also measured in the urine, the spinal fluid, sweat, and saliva.

The most accurate measurement of potassium is total body potassium. The patient lies inside a steel walled room; a nuclear counter is passed over the entire body for 30 minutes and detects the amount of radioactive potassium present (see **Nuclear Scanning**).

Once serum or total body potassium has been determined, a physician can reasonably estimate potassium changes by alterations in the **Electrocardiogram**.

When performed: When there are symptoms of muscle weakness, lethargy, heart rhythm abnormalities, or hormone problems; when patients are taking diuretic drugs; to help determine the source of acidosis, which can cause coma.

Normal values: Potassium levels should range from 4 to 5.5 mEq per liter in serum and 25 to 100 mEq per liter in a 24-hour urine sample.

Abnormal values: Elevated amounts of potassium (hyperkalemia) are found with kidney failure, liver disease, and adrenal cortical hormone deficiency. A large amount of potassium in the blood, usually secondary to kidney failure, can cause the heart to stop beating. Urine levels are most often the opposite of serum levels (high blood potassium with low urine amounts). A few exceptions, however, exist with malabsorption (the potassium is not taken into the bloodstream through the intestines) and with diarrhea.

Serum potassium levels may be decreased in diabetes, vomiting, and diarrhea; from taking laxatives, diuretic drugs, and certain forms of penicillin; with heart rhythm irregularities; and when there is a body magnesium deficiency.

Salivary changes in potassium occur with adrenal disease, and sweat changes occur with certain inherited conditions.

PPD, see *Skin Reaction*

PRA, see *Renin*

PRECIPITIN, see *Complement Fixation*

PRE-EJECTION PERIOD, see *Systolic Time Intervals*

PREGNANCY

Although pregnancy is not really a disease the bodily changes caused by pregnancy are sufficiently complex to be considered a deviation from normal. After fertilization occurs and the fertilized ovum is implanted in the uterus, the mother's body produces a special hormone called human chorionic gonadotropin (HCG). Most pregnancy tests ascertain the presence of HCG in the serum or urine. Formerly, the blood or urine from the patient with suspected pregnancy was injected into a rabbit (A-Z test). If the rabbit's ovaries showed signs of pregnancy, the test was considered positive. The rabbit test is rarely used today; rats, which are easier to obtain than rabbits, have been substituted should this particular version of the test be requested (Friedman).

The newer tests for pregnancy depend on **Agglutination**. Either HCG-sensitized red cells or latex particles (which are treated to act like red blood cells) are added to a patient's serum or urine in a test tube. The pregnant patient has antibodies to chorionic gonadotropin that will react (agglutinate) by clumping together and settling at the bottom of the test tube. The same test may be performed on a slide. When a drop of urine is placed on the slide with sensitizing chemicals, agglutinizing can be seen if pregnancy exists. A slide test takes only two to three minutes and is accurate 96% of the time. These tests are called DAP, Pregnosticon Dri-Dot (or Slide), UCG, and Gravindex, to name a few. Do-it-yourself early pregnancy tests (EPT) are usually slide tests that are very accurate when pregnancy is at least four weeks along but not very accurate when pregnancy is in its very early stage.

The newest test for pregnancy is the Saxena test. It is an extremely sensitive measure of the particular hormone that increases in pregnancy and shows a positive reaction within one week after the patient becomes pregnant. It is especially valuable in detecting ectopic pregnancy (implantation of the fetus outside of the uterus).

When performed: When there is suspicion, or fear, of pregnancy. Pregnancy tests should be routinely performed on all women of child-bearing age (at least from age 12 to age 50) when hospitalized, prior to any X-ray test or treatment or before embarking on any course of drug therapy.

Normal values: A positive test in the presence of pregnancy is normal.

Abnormal values: False positive pregnancy tests may occur when certain hormones are temporarily increased (such as after the menopause); when red blood cells or excessive protein are found in the urine; when certain tranquilizing drugs are taken; and when certain rare uterine and ovarian tumors exist.

PREGNANCY TOXEMIA, see *Rollover*

PREGNOSTICON DRI-DOT (OR SLIDE), see *Pregnancy*

PRESBYOPIA, see *Visual Acuity*

PRISM, see *Strabismus*

PROCTOSIGMOIDOSCOPY, see *Endoscopy*

PROGESTERONE RECEPTOR (PgR), see *Estrogen Receptor*

PROLACTIN

Prolactin (sometimes called lactogenic hormone) is a pituitary hormone that causes the breasts to enlarge and secrete milk. It must be present in order for a mother to nurse her child. In addition, prolactin has been reported to act as a **Growth Hormone** under certain conditions. Blood is taken from a vein and the serum or plasma is tested.

When performed: When a mother who has just given birth is unable to nurse; when certain brain tumors are suspected; when women have menstrual problems.

Normal values: Prolactin levels range from 5 to 25 ng per ml in both men and women but are normally increased in women during pregnancy and while nursing.

Abnormal values: Increased prolactin is found in both men and women during stressful (anxiety-producing) situations; when brain tumors involve the hypothalamus portion of the brain; in certain pituitary tumors (although if the pituitary is destroyed, prolactin levels may be reduced); and in women taking certain drugs—especially those for high blood pressure and some tranquilizers—that may, in turn, cause the breasts to secrete milk without any relation to pregnancy. Prolactin is usually absent when a mother of a newborn is unable to nurse her child.

PROSTATE ENZYME, see *Acid Phosphatase*

PROTEIN-BOUND IODINE, see *Thyroid Function*

PROTEINS, see *Albumin/Globulin*

PROTHROMBIN TIME (Quick Test)

Prothrombin (Factor II) is one of the 12 known factors necessary to stop bleeding (normal body coagulants). Like four other clotting factors, it is manufactured in the liver from vitamin K, which is obtained in the diet primarily from green leafy vegetables, fish, and liver. It is important to know a patient's diet when testing for prothrombin time, since an excess of such foods will alter the test. Coumarin anticoagulant drugs such as warfarin (Coumadin) and dicumarol are often prescribed to prevent thrombophlebitis subsequent to surgery or after an injury. Anticoagulants have, on occasion, also been prescribed after heart attacks and to prevent eye problems in diabetes. They interfere with the liver's ability to make clotting factors.

Although the prothrombin time test indicates the level of prothrombin in the blood, it is more a measure of the overall blood coagulation response to the taking of coumarin anticoagulant drugs. When anticoagulants are given, it may take from three to seven days before the prothrombin time test reflects the drug activity. It is important to know what drugs a patient is taking in addition to anticoagulants before evaluating the prothrombin time. Blood is taken from a vein and the plasma is tested. The test must be performed within an hour after the sample is taken for accurate results, unless the blood sample is immediately frozen.

When performed: Primarily as an indication of the activity of certain anticoagulant drugs (but not heparin); as an indication of how the liver is functioning; as a measure of a patient's dietary intake of vitamin K.

Normal values: Normally it takes 12 to 14 seconds for a fibrin strand (first sign of clotting) to be seen. The test is always run with control plasma that is known to be normal. The result is sometimes reported as the number of seconds it takes a patient's blood to clot compared with the control; more often it is reported as a percentage of the control's plasma prothrombin time compared to patient's prothrombin time, called percentage concentration or percentage of patient's prothrombin activity.

Abnormal values: Any amount of time greater than the control is considered an abnormal value; the longer the patient's prothrombin time in seconds, the lower the percentage of prothrombin activity. When anticoagulants are prescribed, an abnormal value is indicative of the effectiveness of the drug. Ideally, a patient taking a coumarin product should have a prothrombin time two to two and a half times longer than the control, or show between 12% and 20% prothrombin activity.

The prothrombin time is affected when anticoagulants are taken with other drugs. Barbiturates, oral contraceptives, mineral oil, and antacids will shorten the prothrombin time, while aspirin, thyroid hormone, insulin, and oral antidiabetic drugs will lengthen it. It is also prolonged with liver disease; when used for this condition, the test is usually repeated after the patient is given a large amount of vitamin K. Eating large quantities of foods containing vitamin K (salads, fish) will shorten the prothrombin time and require additional anticoagulant drug for effectiveness. Eating commercial French-fried potatoes made with methylpolysiloxane for crispness (the chemical is listed on the label if bought packaged for home use; it is impossible to know about this when dining out) will cause an abnormally decreased prothrombin time for at least a week afterward and could cause a patient to take a dangerous overdose of an anticoagulant drug.

PROTOPORPHYRIN, see *Porphyrin*

PSEUDO-CHOLINESTERASE, see *Cholinesterase*

PSEUDO-GOUT, see *Synovial Fluid*

PSITTACOSIS, see *Complement Fixation*

PSP, see *Phenolsulfonphthalein*

PSYCHOLOGICAL, see *Cornell Index*; *Depression*; *Jenkins Activity Survey*; *Minnesota Multiphasic Personality Inventory*; *Rorschach*; *Thematic Apperception*

PSYCHOLOGICAL HEART DISEASE RISK, see *Jenkins Activity Survey*

PTT, see *Partial Thromboplastin Time*

PULMONARY FUNCTION

Measurements of how well the lungs take in air, how much they can hold, how well they utilize air, and how well they can expel it are important in diagnosing the many different kinds of breathing problems. (The amount of **Oxygen** and **Carbon Dioxide** in the blood are also important measures of the lung's effectiveness.) There are two main types of lung disease. The first type can be caused by loss of lung tissue, inability of the lungs to expand properly, or inability to transfer oxygen to the blood. The second type results from obstruction or narrowing of the main passageways of air (the trachea and bronchial tubes) in the lung.

Most lung function tests are performed by having the patient breathe into a spirometer, an instrument that records the amount of air put through it and the rate of air passage for a specified time. The various tests for pulmonary function are listed and explained below.

Vital capacity (VC), sometimes called forced vital capacity, is probably the most common test of lung volume. It measures how much air the patient can forcefully exhale after inhaling as much air as possible. Usually the body's surface area is calculated and the number is multiplied by 2.5 to obtain the number of liters (a liter approximates a quart) of air that a patient should be able to expel at one time. An average-size 150-pound man should be able to take in and breathe out about 5 liters (5,000 ml) with one forced breath; any amount from 4,000 ml to 6,000 ml is considered within normal limits for men of that size.

Forced expiratory volume (FEV), sometimes called timed vital capacity, is the same as vital capacity with the addition of a time element: the patient is asked to take as deep a breath as possible and then force out the air as hard and as quickly as possible. The amount of air exhaled during the first second of time (FEV_1) is measured. Sometimes measurements of exhalation last for two or three seconds (FEV_2, FEV_3). Normally a person will exhale at least 80% of his vital capacity in the first second and 95% by the third second.

Maximal voluntary ventilation (MVV), sometimes called maximum breathing capacity (MBC), measures the greatest amount of air a person can breathe each minute. The patient is asked to breathe as rapidly and deeply as possible for 15 seconds. The total amount of air exhaled is then multiplied by four, giving the result in liters per minute. The normal amount, like that for the vital capacity, is determined by the individual's body surface area.

Several other measurements may be made of amounts of air the lungs hold. A few of these include the *residual volume* (the air that remains in the lung after the vital capacity is exhaled), the *tidal volume* (how much air is expired with each normal breath), and the *functional residual capacity* (the sum of the last bit of air that can be exhaled during the vital capacity test and the residual volume). These tests are performed by having the patient inhale known amounts of certain gases such as nitrogen and helium and noting which of those gases are absorbed and which are exhaled; they can also be performed with the plethysmograph (a special machine that measures changes in the body's overall volume during breathing; the patient sits in an enclosed controlled-air chamber that resembles a diving bell).

Pulmonary compliance measures how well the lungs can be stretched or distended and then how well they recoil after a full breath; normal is determined by body surface area.

Diffusing capacity shows how well the lungs can transfer oxygen to the blood and eliminate carbon dioxide from the blood at the end points of air passage in the lung (tiny sacs called alveoli). A small amount of carbon monoxide is inhaled and the amount the blood absorbs is measured; normally it should absorb all of it.

Maximum expiratory flow rate (the rate during the middle half of forced vital capacity) and *maximum midexpiratory flow* (the average flow during the middle half of the total expired volume) are two additional measurements used to confirm the results obtained by other tests.

When performed: Whenever there are breathing difficulties such as wheezing, persistent coughing, shortness of breath, repeated episodes of fainting or coma, or difficulties due to exposure to environmental contaminants such as coal dust, asbestos, moldy hay, moldy sugar cane, or compost; when a patient has been working with birds or poultry; following use of certain drugs (especially heroin, methadone, and some antibiotics); with heart failure, chest injuries, and certain nervous system diseases; when there is suspicion of a growth in the lungs; when anxiety causes breathing difficulties; to measure progress in treating lung diseases; to determine when a patient can breathe on his own after being in a mechanical respirator.

Normal values: Most normal values for breathing tests must take into account the age, height and weight (body surface area) and sex of the individual (obviously, the smaller the person, the smaller the lung capacity). After the normal or expected values for a person's size are determined, the measurements are obtained and compared against the standard. A deviation of up to 20% from expected values is considered within normal limits.

Abnormal values: In almost all the pulmonary function tests, results showing a person's breathing or lung capacity to be less than 80% of the expected value (as determined by the person's body surface area) are considered a sign of disease. In general, the tests, when used together, help diagnose restrictive types of lung disease from obstructive types. If the tests show abnormal results, the normal procedure is to administer a bronchodilator drug such as isoetharine (usually by inhalation) and then repeat the measurements; if the drug produces bronchodilatation and causes marked improvement, the lung disease is usually considered reversible. For example, with asthma the vital capacity will increase after a bronchodilator drug; with emphysema there will be no improvement. The vital capacity measurement is reduced with nerve diseases that affect respiratory muscles (Guillain-Barré disease, myasthenia gravis), edema of the lungs, and conditions that take up space in the lung area such as tumors.

The other lung function tests will give less than predicted results depending on the specific cause of the disease and the extent of the disease process. In chronic bronchitis (an obstructive type of disease) the vital capacity and the

FEV₁ are reduced. In sarcoidosis (where the lung alveoli, which transfer oxygen to the bloodstream, are thickened), the FEV_1 is usually normal because there is no obstruction to the bronchial tubes. The lungs will not recoil normally with emphysema.

PULSE ANALYSIS

The word "pulse" refers to the sudden expansion of the walls of a blood vessel as the blood is forced through it by the heartbeat. The carotid pulse is measured by placing a sensitive recording instrument on the side of the neck over the area of the carotid artery. It specifically reflects the action of the valve from the heart to the aorta (the left side of the heart). The jugular vein pulse is measured by placing the recording instrument over the area where the vein pulsations are most visible (usually just above the collarbone). It is a measure of the effectiveness of the right side of the heart.

When performed: The carotid artery pulse is measured to confirm already suspected aortic heart valve disease (on the left side of the heart, which pumps blood to the body). The jugular vein pulse is measured to ascertain the function of the right side of the heart (which pumps blood to the lungs), including the right-sided heart valves. It is also used to confirm pericardial disease. (The pericardium is the sac around the heart; it can fill up with fluid or tighten around the heart and impair heart function.)

Normal values: The two pulse impulses form standard recorded wave patterns (much as the standard electroencephalogram) and are interpreted by a physician.

Abnormal values: Variations from the normal wave patterns reveal specific heart disease conditions.

PUPILLARY REFLEX

The pupils of the eye (the openings in the center surrounded by the colored iris) open and close (widen and narrow) when exposed to different amounts of light and when focusing on near or far objects. The smaller the opening, the more clearly objects can be seen at different distances (in photography this is called "depth of field"). To test pupillary reflexes, first, a strong light is directed into the eye to note the pupil's reaction; second, the patient is asked to look at objects both close up and far away and the pupil is observed.

When performed: Whenever brain, nerve, or eye disease is suspected; whenever certain drug abuse or overdose is suspected.

Normal values: Normally, when a bright light is directed toward the eye (or when a person is in bright sunlight), the pupils contract and become very small (miosis). As the amount of light diminishes, the pupils widen. When a person looks at an object close up, the pupils usually contract (accommodation). If light is directed to one eye only, normally the pupil of the other eye also becomes smaller, even if it is blocked off from the light source. As people become older, pupil size normally becomes smaller. Both pupils should be round and of the same size.

Abnormal values: In patients with Argyll-Robertson pupil, light will not diminish pupil size, but looking at a close object will. The condition is most often a result of syphilis. In patients who are blind in one eye, the pupil may still respond to light in the other eye, but not to direct light. When the pupil does not react at all, it is usually indicative of nerve-brain disease. Various drugs can cause either sustained dilatation or contraction of the pupil. Narcotic drugs usually cause fixed "pinpoint" pupils.

PURE TONE, see *Hearing Function*

PUTATIVE PARENT, see *Disputed Parentage*

PYELOGRAM, see *Radiography*

PYRIDOXINE (Vitamin B6)

Vitamin B6 (also called pyridoxine) is essential to the metabolism of proteins, carbohydrates, fats, and fatty acids. Brewer's yeast, black strap molasses, bran, and organ meats contain large amounts of pyridoxine. Vitamin B6 deficiency is rare but is seen in pregnancy and with the ingestion of certain drugs (isoniazid, penicillamine). Symptoms of deficiency include dermatitis, conjunctivitis, neuritis, loss of appetite, nausea, vomiting, and lethargy. In addition, B6 deficiency can cause anemias and oxalate crystals in urine. The urine is usually examined for the amount of pyridoxal (the active metabolic product of pyridoxine, which is easier to measure). A 24-hour urine specimen is required.

When performed: When symptoms indicate a possible deficiency of vitamin B6.

Normal values: Excretion of 35 to 55 mcg of pyridoxal per day in the urine is considered normal.

Abnormal values: Excretion of less than 35 mcg of pyridoxal per day is indicative of deficiency.

Q-FEVER, see *Agglutination*

QUICK, see *Prothrombin Time*

QUIZ ELECTROCARDIOGRAM, see *Electrocardiogram*

RADARKYMOGRAM

Radarkymography is considered one of the best tests for delineating the outer borders of the heart. It is noninvasive (requiring no penetration into the body or direct contact with the heart) and therefore much safer than invasive tests. Moreover, a permanent graphic illustration of the results is provided by means of videotape recording apparatus. Electrical impulses, similar to radar waves, are projected over the chest and then picked up by a radar tracking instrument. These are then transposed on a fluoroscope to show heart size and shape. The test can be performed on very ill patients who cannot be moved or who cannot stand in front of an X-ray machine. It is quite similar to, and often used in place of, cineangiography, which provides X-ray motion pictures of dye injected into the heart (an invasive procedure).

When performed: The test is performed primarily to study the physical characteristics of heart muscle contractions, especially in very sick patients. It is also used when aortic disease is suspected or when aneurysm (a weakened area of the muscle wall that balloons out) of heart muscle is being considered.

Normal values: Certain standard waves (based on thousands of test recordings of normal hearts) represent the normal, expected heart contraction.

Abnormal values: Abnormal waves are noted during heart contraction with certain heart valve diseases that cause bulging of the heart muscle and with weakening of the heart walls or the walls of the aorta as it leaves the heart.

RADIOACTIVE IODINE SCREENING, see *Thyroid Function*

RADIOALLERGOSORBENT, see *RAST*

RADIOGRAPHY

Radiography, or the use of X-rays, is an integral part of many different testing procedures. A chest X-ray for a cough, for instance, is no different from a screening blood test for anemia or infection; it may not always reveal a specific disease, but it offers clues toward a diagnosis. Much depends on the type of X-ray. There are X-rays of specific parts of the body or specific organs taken from different angles. There are X-rays using a contrast dye (usually an iodine solution) that cannot be penetrated and that causes great contrast on the X-ray film, silhouetting or imaging whatever tissue the dye fills; the dye reveals organs that normally would not be seen by X-ray alone. The dye may also be used to show concentration in an organ or to follow how efficiently and rapidly an organ eliminates that dye (excretion test).

An X-ray of a bone will show if that bone is broken (or has a slight crack) and thus is essentially a test for fracture. The chest X-ray will show any pathology in the lung as well as the size, shape, and position of the heart and, like the standard electrocardiogram, will help diagnose suspected heart problems; in this sense it is a "test" for coronary disease. A fluoroscopic examination will show heart movement (using X-rays) and, with the use of a contrast dye, will delineate just what happens when a person swallows; the contrast dye outlines the stomach, the intestines, and the large bowel. The gall bladder, joint cavities, the spinal canal, the uterus and tubes, the lungs, and even arteries and veins are also outlined by contrast dye.

Angiography is the particular study of the arterial blood vessels by X-rays and contrast media. In cerebral angiography, the dye is injected into the neck arteries and X-ray pictures are taken of the circulation of the brain. (The dye fills and outlines arteries that normally cannot be visualized by X-ray.) Coronary angiography is similar, except that the dye is injected into the coronary arteries (those that feed heart muscle) via a catheter (thin tube) from the arm or neck through the heart into the aorta; the dye is specifically placed to fill the tiny arteries that supply the heart, the plugging of which seems to cause most heart attacks.

Venography is similar to angiography except that the dye is injected into a vein instead of an artery. This test is especially valuable for detecting thrombophlebitis (a clot blocking the passage of blood in a vein, usually—but not always—existing along with an infectious process). There are many newer tests to detect thrombosis (using sound waves or air pressure measurements); however, phlebography (X-rays of dye in the vein) is still considered the most accurate for blood clots in veins. Normally no clot or blockage is seen in veins.

Pyelography (intravenous pyelography, or IVP) is the study of the kidney, ureters, and bladder by X-rays and contrast media. When the contrast dye is injected into the bloodstream (usually through an arm vein), it will almost immediately concentrate in the kidneys and then pass down into the bladder. Normally the dye shows in the kidney within minutes and assumes an expected silhouette. If cysts, tumors, or other diseases are present, the dye will take longer to appear and abnormal filling defects will be seen. In special circumstances, the dye is injected directly into the kidney arteries (usually by catheters inserted into leg arteries and then pushed up to kidney level) to determine if both kidney arteries are of normal size and shape and are not narrowed or blocked. This is called a renal arteriography test and is particularly useful in cases of undiagnosed high blood pressure.

The same test can be performed by inserting a contrast dye through a cystoscope into the urethra and then via tiny tubes into the ureters and watching the dye fill up in the kidneys; it is called retrograde pyelography. This form of the test is usually used when there is some doubt about kidney function and when the cause of the problem is thought to be below the kidneys.

Oral cholecystography, using X-rays and contrast media, will detect gall stones (a plain X-ray of the liver and gall bladder area usually will not). The patient follows his usual diet for several days prior to the test; at dinner the night before and breakfast just prior to the test no fat is ingested. The patient takes special dye tablets the night before. If the bile ducts and gall bladder are normal, the X-ray (taken the next morning) will show the gall bladder filled with the dye. The patient is then given a fatty meal to eat; X-rays are taken every 15 minutes afterward to determine if emptying of the gall bladder is normal. If stones are present, they usually are seen in contrast to the dye. If the gall bladder does not fill up with the dye the next morning, the test is usually repeated with a double dose of the dye tablets before the results are considered abnormal. An abnormal test can mean gall stones, but it can also mean a sluggish or infected gall bladder or liver disease.

Cholangiography, sometimes called intravenous cholangiography (IVC), is another test of the functioning of the ducts that carry bile from the liver to the gall bladder and then to the intestine. It is usually employed when two oral cholecystography tests fail to show the gall bladder, or after a patient has had gall bladder surgery and still has symptoms. The dye is injected into an arm vein; X-ray pictures are taken every 15 minutes (usually for an hour) until the bile ducts and the gall bladder can be visualized. It is especially valuable when a gall stone is suspected in a bile duct rather than in the gall bladder. Occasionally this test too must be performed a second time in order to find the gall stone or to ascertain that the gall bladder is not functioning.

Transhepatic cholangiography may be performed when it is impossible to tell whether jaundice is caused by bile stones or by liver damage. A needle is inserted into the liver and after a bile duct is located, dye is injected directly into the duct. If the liver is not outlined by the dye, bile stone blockage is indicated and surgery is usually performed immediately to remove the obstruction.

A *gastrointestinal (GI) series*, or contrast radiography of the gastrointestinal tract, can consist of many different tests. The patient may swallow a mouthful of barium (a compound that resists X-rays and shows up in marked contrast on the X-ray film). As the barium passes down the esophagus into the stomach, the size, shape, and activity of the esophagus can be observed through fluoroscopic examination. When sufficient barium is ingested to fill the stomach, it can be seen both by fluoroscopic examination and by X-ray pictures. Any filling "defect" (a place where the normal outline of barium should be seen but is not) is usually an indication of disease (ulcer, growth, or infection). When barium is in the stomach, it is common to tilt the patient so that his head is lower than his feet; the procedure helps to diagnose a hiatal hernia (a weakness of the lower end of the esophagus and the diaphragm around the esophagus), which can cause consistent heartburn. The barium is then followed into the upper (small) intestines where the physician searches for other defects. Sufficient barium is usually given to outline the entire small intestine.

To test for disease in the large intestine (the colon and rectum), barium is usually instilled by enema until the lower bowel is filled. Again, defects in places where barium should normally be seen can indicate disease. In contrast, visible pouches of barium can indicate polyps. After the barium is expelled, X-rays are again taken to see if any residual barium has been captured by the bowel; this can also indicate a disease process (at times additional air is introduced to exaggerate the contrast). If a complete gastrointestinal series is to be performed, the barium enema is given first. A barium enema can also help prevent unnecessary surgery for appendicitis by revealing the cause of abdominal pain.

Arthrography refers to X-rays of the joints using a contrast media (dye) or air to outline the joint spaces. Arthrography may be performed on almost any joint. Most frequently the knee is examined, in order to diagnose meniscal injury. (Menisci are the small cartilage cushions in the knee joint that separate the bones of the upper and lower leg.) Fluoroscopy is used after the dye is injected to help locate the area to be studied; then X-ray films are taken.

In *myelography*, sometimes called a myelogram test, contrast dye is injected into the spinal canal (using the **Cerebrospinal Fluid** test technique), in order to study the bones of the spinal column (almost always the lower, or lumbar, spinal column) and especially the spaces, or discs, between the bones. Usually the patient is placed on a special table so that his position can be changed to distribute the dye better and, of even greater importance, so that as much of the dye as possible can be withdrawn at the end of the test. If it is not possible to withdraw all the dye, the removal technique is repeated the following day.

In *bronchography* contrast media are dropped into the lungs through a catheter (tiny tube) inserted into the trachea in order to examine the bronchial tubes—their size (opening), location, and number. The technique, though not in frequent use, is still a fairly definitive test for bronchiectasis (abnormally dilated passages of the bronchial tubes).

Hysterosalpingography is a test to discover whether the fallopian tubes are open to allow passage of the egg or ovum from the ovary to the uterus. It is one of many fertility tests conducted when a couple is unable to have children (see **Rubin**). The tubes may be closed as a result of infection (appendicitis, gonorrhea) or other disease or abnormally located uterine tissue.

Pneumoencephalography (PEG) is a test to outline the cerebrospinal fluid spaces within the brain. Sterile air or a gas is injected into the spinal column (using the **Cerebrospinal Fluid** test technique) and rises up to the brain area, replacing the fluid normally present and giving a clear outline of the spaces, called ventricles. Should defects be seen (such as a suspected tumor or loss of brain substance), the patient may be moved about to provide better visualization.

At times a cisternal puncture is used instead of the usual cerebrospinal fluid tap in the lower spine, usually when the patient has a vertebral defect. With the cisternal puncture, the needle is inserted at the base of the skull just above the first vertebrae. **Computerized Tomography** is being used as a less dangerous substitute for this particular test.

Lymphangiography is a test to determine the effectiveness of the lymph vessels and lymph glands (lymph is a transparent fatty fluid that goes from body tissues back into the bloodstream). When lymph vessels become obstructed or inoperative, edema (water retention) usually results; cancer tends to be spread via the lymph system. Dye is slowly injected into the lymph vessels to be studied, and the patient is X-rayed at that time and then again in 24 hours.

Mammography is the use of X-rays to visualize breast tissue (mammary glands), primarily to detect a growth and secondarily to distinguish, when possible, a malignant from a benign growth. The test is usually performed prior to any breast surgery and especially on women over the age of 30 who have a family history of breast cancer. Usually, the breast is X-rayed from the top and from the side. Xeromammography is a special X-ray technique that is said to provide greater detail with less X-ray exposure. Many physicians feel the danger of too much X-ray makes this test unsatisfactory. While breast X-rays have some advocates, it is a fact that many "masses" detected through these processes are not always cancer and that one out of five "lumps" are not detected.

Tomography (not to be confused with **Computerized Tomography**) is a special radiographic technique of focusing the X-ray on a specific thin-layer cross section of the body so as to accentuate the details of that plane of tissue.

Note: Any radiography test using a contrast dye may cause a reaction in a patient—from minor itching and a rash to a fatality. The patient must always be screened to rule out any allergy to the dye. Patients with known allergic diseases such as asthma must be tested with extreme caution.

As with many medical decisions, the risks of testing must be weighed against the benefits. Too much X-ray exposure may well cause a problem worse than the suspected disease for which the patient is being tested. Whether the benefits of testing outweigh the hazards is something that must be decided between the patient and his physician after a full and frank discussion.

The newest form of radiography is the Dynamic Spatial Reconstructor (DSR) that utilizes a great many X-ray tubes in a half circle around the patient; each X-ray detected by a television receiver opposite it. This device allows three-dimensional images of organs in motion, such as the heart beating or the lung breathing.

When performed: In general, radiography is performed to detect any disease process that cannot be diagnosed by other means. Specific indications are discussed in the descriptions of the procedures above.

Normal values: Each area of the body has a standard photographic pattern. Through training and experience the physician can determine whether the patterns seen on an X-ray (including minor variations for individual patients) are normal.

Abnormal values: The finding of suggested pathology or the absence of an

X-ray shadow that should be visible is considered abnormal, as described in the various procedures.

RADIOIMMUNOASSAY, see *Nuclear Scanning*

RADIOIMMUNOSORBENT, see *RAST*

RADIOISOTOPE SCANNING, see *Nuclear Scanning*

RADIONUCLIDE, see *Nuclear Scanning*

RAPE, see *Semen*

RAPID PLASMA REAGIN (RPR), see *Syphilis*

RAST

Although skin tests (see **Skin Reaction**) are still the most common way to test for allergy, the newest technique for measuring a potential allergic reaction is called the RAST test (sometimes called radioimmunosorbent assay test or radioallergosorbent test). It begins as a generalized measurement of a patient's serum immunoglobulin E, or IgE (see **Immunoglobulin**), which will react to known allergy-causing substances (grasses, foods, cosmetics, animal hairs, etc.). The test is a form of Coombs' test reaction (see **Agglutination**). If a patient's blood contains antibodies to certain allergy-provoking substances, these antibodies will combine with known nuclear-radiolabeled allergens and can be so detected.

A positive RAST test (one that shows a reaction) is really a qualitative measure of IgE in the body; the test not only detects the allergens but can also show how much of an allergen it takes to cause an allergic manifestation (asthma, hay fever, eczema). The RAST test is much less time-consuming (one day versus several months), less painful (one needleprick versus scores), and less dangerous (no chance of severe allergic reactions) for a patient than the skin-scratch tests for allergy.

Blood is taken from a vein and the serum is examined. Usually the serum is tested against specific groups of known allergy-causing antigens (such as all the grasses and trees and various weeds, animals, and house dust mites). When a grouping shows a positive reaction, further tests are performed on individual items in that group if known antibodies are available (not all known antibodies have been processed into allergens for testing).

When performed: To help find the specific cause of an allergy; as a means of measuring progress in the treatment of allergies.

Normal values: A RAST negative reaction indicates that no allergenic antibodies are present.

Abnormal values: A RAST positive reaction, especially in the presence of high serum IgE levels, indicates the presence of allergenic antibodies. Sometimes a positive test is reported as from class I to class IV, the latter indicating a very large amount of antibodies. Because different laboratories may show different results (some will report a positive reaction where others report negative), it is usual to have RAST tests repeated by more than one laboratory.

RAT-BITE FEVER, see *Agglutination*

RBC, see *Red Blood Cell*

RECTILINEAR SCAN, see *Nuclear Scanning*

RED BLOOD CELL

The red blood cells (erythrocytes) contain hemoglobin (about 60% of the body's iron), which is the essential carrier of oxygen in the blood. Beside carrying oxygen to all parts of the body, red blood cells pick up certain waste products (such as carbon dioxide) that are given off later by the lungs. In testing, the red blood cells are counted as well as stained to reveal the size, shape, and hemoglobin content. Sickle cells are seen directly this way, as are certain anemias (see **Blood Cell Differential**). Blood taken from a vein is most commonly used; a drop of blood, usually from the fingertip or earlobe, can also be collected. The blood is viewed through the microscope and counted manually or by automated machines.

When performed: When there is suspicion of one of the anemias or polycythemia (a disease where the bone marrow makes too many red blood cells); in certain parasitic diseases; to verify certain poisonings; to help determine blood loss after hemorrhage.

Normal values: Normal levels for men range from 4 to 6 million red cells per cubic millimeter (cu mm) of blood. Women may have a slightly lower count, and newborn babies a higher count.

Abnormal values: Higher than normal values are usually found with polycythemia, dehydration, certain kidney diseases, and lung conditions where there is difficulty in breathing and the body needs more oxygen. Lower than normal values are usually found with anemias, severe infections, certain cancers, **Malaria**, lead poisoning, and after prolonged bleeding.

RED BLOOD CELL ENZYME SCREENING, see *Glucose 6-Phosphate Dehydrogenase*

RED BLOOD CELL HEMOLYSIS, see *Haptoglobin*; *Tocopherols*

RED BLOOD CELL INDICES

New electronic equipment has made determination of the red blood cell (erythrocyte) indices a valuable aid not only in classifying anemia but in determining the basic cause of the anemia and in helping to decide the specific therapy. The three indices are (1) mean corpuscular volume (MCV), a ratio of the hematocrit to the red blood cell count, expressed as the area of cubic microns (cu μ) per cell; (2) mean corpuscular hemoglobin (MCH), a ratio of the hemoglobin to the red blood cell count, expressed as picograms (pg) of hemoglobin per cell; and (3) mean corpuscular hemoglobin concentration (MCHC), a ratio of hemoglobin to hematocrit, expressed as a percentage. (See **Hematocrit**; **Hemoglobin**; **Red Blood Cell**.) Blood is taken from a vein (or from a fingertip, earlobe, or heel) and placed in a special indices chamber.

When performed: When the cause or type of anemia cannot be determined; after the cause of an anemia is determined, to follow the progress of therapy; in certain cases of liver disease and suspected vitamin deficiencies.

Normal values: Normal levels for MCV range from 83 to 103 cu μ; for MCH, from 27 to 35 pg; for MCHC, from 32% to 36%.

Abnormal values: The MCH and MCV are lowered with some genetically caused anemias and with iron deficiency, liver disease, and blood loss. The MCHC is increased with anemias due to inadequate blood formation. The MCV and MCHC are increased with pernicious anemia, tapeworm infestation, and when taking certain medicines.

REFLEX

A reflex test is a measure of the reaction of the body to stimulation. Most commonly muscles are measured for their reflex reaction. Testing for the reflex reaction of the eyelid, the cornea (surface of the eye over the iris and lens), the pupils (see **Pupillary Reflex**), and the skin surface can help in the diagnosis of disease. (See **Caloric** test for ear reflex responses.)

In general, a muscle is tested by applying sufficient pressure to cause stretching of its fibers. In the knee-jerk reflex test, for example, the tapping of the patellar tendon (usually with a rubber hammer) just below the kneecap stretches the attached thigh muscle that lifts the lower leg. The muscle reacts by contracting (shortening) and the lower leg lifts suddenly and involuntarily.

Arm and leg muscle reflex tests are called "deep" reflex tests because of the force of the tap necessary to elicit a response. When a reflex is tested by a gentle stroking motion over or near the muscle, it is called a "superficial" reflex test. For example, when the upper abdomen is stroked, the stomach muscles contract and pull the umbilicus (navel) upward. If a gentle stroke is applied just inside the upper thigh, adjacent to the testicle, the scrotum (the sac that holds the testicle) will suddenly rise upward on the same side that is stroked because of contraction of the cremasteric muscle.

Virtually every muscle can be tested this way, but only about a dozen reflex tests are routinely performed. Each muscle reflex represents an area of the spinal cord where the nerves to that muscle arise and, of course, the nerve itself. Thus testing for a specific muscle reflex can determine the exact area of the nervous system involved. For example, the bicep (the usually large, bulging muscle of the upper arm) is activated by nerves that come from between the fifth and sixth cervical vertebrae (the neck bones of the spine).

Failure to elicit the reflex, or an extremely exaggerated reflex, indicates disease of the nerve from the muscle to the spinal cord, disease of the spinal cord itself, or disease of the nerves from the spinal cord. The knee-jerk reflex is indicative of nerves that come from the lumbar (lower back) portion of the spine. Superficial reflexes also indicate nervous system locations. Pathology in certain nerves that come directly from the brain can be determined by the corneal reflex. When the colored part of the eye is touched with a piece of cotton, both eyes should immediately close as a reflex action. Failure of the eyes to close, or only one eye closing (either the same side or the opposite), indicates disease inside the brain.

The usual instrument for testing reflexes is the rubber hammer, but the edge of the hand will do as well. When it seems impossible to obtain a positive reflex reaction, the patient may be asked to perform some other muscular act to draw attention away from the area being tested. This will relax the muscle and allow a normal reflex. To obtain a knee-jerk reaction, for example, the physician may ask the patient to interlock his fingers and pull hard with both hands.

When performed: As part of a routine physical examination to ascertain the functioning of nerves, muscles, and spinal cord; whenever nerve, muscle, or brain damage is suspected; after any injury.

Normal values: Pressure or stimulus on any relaxed muscle should cause a contraction of that muscle, or at least a reaction indicating that the pressure or stimulus was acknowledged by the body. Experience has taught doctors the expected responses so that weak or overly strong reactions can be noted. The reflexes on exact opposite sides or parts of the body should be about the same.

Reflex reactions are usually recorded on a "plus" scale from 1 to 4: 4-plus means hyperactive; 1-plus means weak or inadequate; 2-plus and 3-plus are average.

Abnormal values: Total absence of a reflex or extreme hyperactivity is considered abnormal. Specific pathological reflexes include the Babinski, in which stroking the sole of the foot causes the toes to point up and separate (normally the toes turn down as a response). The reaction is indicative of brain disease. The abnormal doll's-eye reflex occurs when the head is rotated from side to side and the eyes follow the movement to each side (normally they continue to look straight ahead). This is indicative of severe brain disease, but it can also occur with a large overdose of barbiturate drugs.

Note: The Bender-Purdue reflex test, sometimes called the symmetric tonic neck reflex test, is performed primarily to determine whether an infant will hold his head up high and look forward and up when creeping. The position and use of the arms, hands, knees, and feet are also recorded. The manner of the child's movements is said to be indicative of the child's ability to learn (to be educated).

REFRACTION, see *Visual Acuity*

RENAL ARTERIOGRAPHY, see *Radiography*

RENAL STONE, see *Urinary Tract Calculus*

RENIN

Renin is an enzyme produced by the kidney. (A renin-type substance that acts exactly like renin is also produced by the liver as an adverse reaction when oral contraceptive drugs or other female hormones are taken.) Renin regulates the production of the hormone **Aldosterone**, which in turn controls the salt and water balance in the body. It also metabolizes to form other compounds that cause the muscles around arteries to tighten and become smaller in size, thus raising the blood pressure.

The test is really a renin activity measurement, since an angiotensin compound made from renin is actually measured (see **Rollover**). It is important to know how much salt the patient has been eating for at least three days prior to the test (the less salt, the higher the renin values). The patient should be lying down for several hours before the test (standing and even sitting increases renin activity). Usually blood is taken from a vein and the plasma is tested. It is now becoming common to measure renin activity separately in each of the kidney veins, since the comparative values are important in evaluating the potential success of kidney surgery as a treatment for high blood pressure.

When performed: To diagnose one cause of high blood pressure and to help ascertain the type of therapy and whether that therapy will be effective; when adrenal disease is suspected.

Normal values: Plasma renin activity (PRA) measures from 0.2 to 4 ng per ml per hour, depending on the amount of salt in the diet and for how long the patient was in an upright position before the test. Normal values are higher in the early morning hours. When renin activity is measured in each of the kidney veins, there should be no significant difference between the left and right vein.

Abnormal values: PRA is increased with high blood pressure caused by kidney disease, sometimes with chronic kidney disease alone, following kidney injury, with certain adrenal tumors, and with chronic liver disease. Increased values can also occur with pregnancy, with certain diuretic drugs, and with a salt-free diet. Values are usually decreased when patients are eating large amounts of salt or foods containing salt, when patients are taking certain steroid hormone drugs, when the adrenal glands secrete excessive aldosterone, and when high blood pressure comes from eating large amounts of licorice.

RENOGRAM, see *Nuclear Scanning*

RESIDUAL LUNG VOLUME, see *Pulmonary Function*

RETICULOCYTE COUNT

Reticulocytes are immature red blood cells. The reticulocyte count is a measurement (though not precise) of the production of erythrocytes (red blood cells). When the production of erythrocytes is increased by a process that stimulates bone marrow, the reticulocyte count also increases. Any bodily process that can limit red blood cell production (infection, renal disease) can limit the number of reticulocytes in the blood. A drop of blood is stained, and the reticulocytes are viewed under the microscope and counted.

When performed: To evaluate the patient's response to therapy for anemia and polycythemia (an excessive amount of red blood cells).

Normal values: The reticulocyte count is reported as a proportion of the red blood cell count. The usual range is 0.5 to 1.5 reticulocytes per 100 red blood cells.

Abnormal values: The reticulocyte count is decreased in severe autoimmune types of hemolytic (blood-cell-destroying) disease. The count is increased when bone marrow cells are made more active (as with recovery from anemia or following hemorrhage).

RETINOL (Vitamin A)

Deficiency of vitamin A (a fat-soluble alcohol) is considered a major problem of nutrition. Usually vitamin A is supplied in minimal amounts in the average diet. It is found mostly in fish and fish oils, dairy products, eggs, green and yellow vegetables, and polar bear liver. Some health faddists who eat excessive amounts of foods high in vitamin A may display symptoms of hair loss, fatigue, irritability, cerebral edema, and yellowish skin color.

Vitamin A deficiency is a major cause of blindness in young children in parts of the world where the diet is inadequate. Night blindness and "dry eye" are early indications of the deficiency. Blood is taken from a vein and the vitamin A, retinol, or carotene (forms of the vitamin) is measured from the serum. Retinol can also be measured from a liver **Biopsy**.

When performed: With vision problems, especially inability to see at night; when there are teeth and bone growth problems; in certain cases of sterility; with children who are extremely irritable with no obvious cause.

Normal values: Serum levels of 30 to 60 mcg per 100 ml or more are indicative of adequate storage and intake of vitamin A.

Abnormal values: Less than 20 mcg per 100 ml indicates decreased absorption of vitamin A, retinol, or carotene and may be found with food absorption problems such as pancreatic and biliary insufficiency, celiac disease (in addition to the associated eye problems), sprue, and excessive use of mineral oil as a laxative. Some patients with vitamin A deficiency have impaired senses of taste and smell. Patients who take oral contraceptives may have increased serum levels of vitamin A.

Note: The vitamin A tolerance test consists of giving a patient a large dose of vitamin A by mouth and measuring serum levels four to five hours later. Normally vitamin A levels will rise to greater than 150 mcg per 100 ml. Failure to rise indicates improper fat absorption by the intestine.

RETINOSCOPY, see *Visual Acuity*

RETROGRADE PYELOGRAPHY, see *Radiography*

RH FACTOR, see *Agglutination*

RIBOFLAVIN (Vitamin B$_2$)

Deficiency of vitamin B$_2$, or riboflavin, can cause many eye problems (ulceration, cataracts, corneal vascularization, burning and itching) and skin problems (scaling, inflammation), as well as problems in the blood (leucocytopenia, granulocytopenia) and the nervous system (neuritis). Riboflavin is found mostly in milk, meat, and nuts. It can be measured in both the urine and the blood.

When performed: With skin, eye, and nervous system problems that cannot be diagnosed.

Normal values: Normal urinary riboflavin excretion is from 30 to 100 mcg in a 6-hour sample. In the blood riboflavin should be greater than 15 mcg per 100 ml of red blood cells.

Abnormal values: Less than 30 mcg in the urine or less than 15 mcg in the blood is indicative of sufficient deficiency to cause symptoms.

RINGWORM, see *Fungus*

RINNE, see *Tuning Fork*

RISK FACTOR FOR HEART DISEASE, see *Jenkins Activity Survey*

RKG, see *Radarkymogram*

ROBINSON-POWER-KEPLER, see *Chloride*

ROLLOVER

Toxemia of pregnancy (more correctly referred to as pregnancy-induced hypertension, since no "toxin" is involved) is probably the most serious side effect of having a child. It usually develops during the last three months of pregnancy and, unless it is detected at its earliest stage, it can be fatal to both mother and child. Until the rollover test was devised, there was no easy way to determine which women were more susceptible than others to toxemia. While the test is not considered perfect at this time, it is the best available. The patient lies on her left side and the blood pressure is tested. Then the patient rolls over on her back and the blood pressure is measured immediately and then again five minutes later. The test seems to be an indication of a pregnant woman's susceptibility to producing angiotensin, an enzyme made in the kidney that can cause high blood pressure (see **Renin** test).

When performed: On all pregnant women, especially those having their first baby; on a regular basis after the third month of pregnancy.

Normal values: The blood pressure readings should not change after the patient rolls over.

Abnormal values: An increase in the diastolic blood pressure, usually by more than 20 mm Hg (see **Blood Pressure**), within five minutes of rolling over is considered a warning sign; the pregnant patient is then watched far more closely for blood pressure changes.

ROMBERG, see *Caloric*

ROPES, see *Synovial Fluid*

RORSCHACH

The Rorschach test, invented by a Swiss psychiatrist, consists of a series of essentially formless black inkblots (some also containing red spots), which a subject is asked to interpret. Rorschach believed that personality traits could be revealed by the way a person reacted to these abstract shapes. The Rorschach test is scored on the basis of several criteria: whether all or only part of the inkblot is used in description; whether the subject goes into unusual detail (compulsive personalities supposedly respond first to details instead of the overall blot); whether form or color is more important (people who are upset by color are supposed to be more emotional); and whether motion is read into the blot (human movement is supposed to represent creativeness). Many uncommon responses are assumed to indicate a schizophrenic disturbance.

Rorschach "scores" have demonstrated little validity as indicators of individual behavior and personality. When the test is used by a therapist to help form hypotheses about an individual, there is the danger that the therapist will make highly personalized interpretations that cannot be considered scientifically valid.

The Holtzman inkblot technique is a similar test using different types of blots. The Holtzman allows the subject to give only one response to the inkblot (in the Rorschach a patient is asked to give as many interpretations of the blot as possible).

When performed: The test is performed ostensibly to aid in the diagnosis of neurotic or mentally disturbed persons. It is usually given as a part of a battery of tests, since recent studies have cast doubt on the value of Rorschach test interpretations for either diagnosis or prognosis.

Normal values: There are certain standard responses to the inkblots that a majority of subjects state.

Abnormal values: In people who are clearly suffering from mental problems, peculiar responses verify the obvious.

ROSE SHEEP CELL AGGLUTINATION, see *Agglutination*

ROUTINE URINALYSIS, see *Urine Examination*

RUBELLA, see *Agglutination*

RUBIN

The Rubin test is one of several tests performed in cases of infertility. Specifically, it determines whether the fallopian tubes (which carry the ovum, or egg, from the ovary to the uterus) are open or blocked. Carbon dioxide gas is forced into the uterus under pressure; if the tubes are normal (open), the gas is detected in the abdomen. Occasionally the test procedure itself acts therapeutically to open blocked tubes.

When performed: When disease of the fallopian tubes is suspected; in cases of sterility.

Normal values: Normally the carbon dioxide passes easily through the tubes into the abdomen.

Abnormal values: Obstruction of the fallopian tubes may occur in endometriosis and infections (particularly following previous delivery or abortion) or following peritoneal inflammation (appendicitis). Occasionally the patient may have a spasm of the tubes during the test, giving a false negative result. Therefore, if the test is negative (tubes blocked), a second test should be performed for verification.

RUMPEL-LEEDE, see *Capillary Fragility*

SALICYLATES

A salicylate is any salt of salicylic acid (prepared synthetically or obtained from wintergreen leaves or the bark of white birch). Aspirin is one of the most common sources of salicylates as are many other drugs used to minimize pain. Taking an excessive amount causes poisoning. Aspirin is often added to chickenfeed to ease the pain and discomfort of chickens that are bred in crowded conditions. Aspirin also seems to increase the amount of fat in chickens. Eating large quantities of chicken that have been fed aspirin can increase the blood salicylate level. Blood is taken from a vein for testing. Urine may be tested for screening to consider salicylate poisoning.

When performed: When patients are taking large doses of salicylates for arthritis or rheumatic fever; in cases of suspected accidental aspirin poisoning in children; in coma.

Normal values: Normally there are no salicylates in the blood or urine. Therapeutic levels of salicylates in the blood range from 5 to 12 mg per 100 ml.

Abnormal values: More than 30 mg per 100 ml in the blood is considered toxic. Symptoms of salicylate poisoning include dizziness, nausea, vomiting, tinnitus (ringing in the ears), restlessness, disorientation, rapid breathing, shock, and coma. Salicylate poisoning can also cause abnormally low blood sugar levels.

SALT LOADING, see *Aldosterone*

SARCOIDOSIS, see *Kveim*

SAXENA, see *Pregnancy*

THE ENCYCLOPEDIA OF

SCABIES INFESTATION

Scabies is a dermatological condition caused by a biting, burrowing mite. The incidence of scabies is increasing greatly, even among people who keep themselves fastidiously clean. A skin test in which extracts of the mite are injected is the primary method of differentiating between scabies and other dermatological conditions. Another test is to paint the skin with fluorescein dye and then shine ultraviolet light over the area; the burrowing tunnels then fluoresce. Serum immunoglobulin A is reduced in patients with scabies (see **Immunoglobulin**).

When performed: To differentiate certain rash-causing itching patterns from syphilis or lice infestations; whenever venereal disease is suspected; when a woman has a dermatitis of the nipples or a man has a rash over his scrotum; when a patient has a localized rash over the buttocks.

Normal values: There should be no evidence of the mite on direct examination and no reaction to the skin test.

Abnormal values: A positive skin test reaction (a hard, red nodule forms) confirms the diagnosis of scabies.

SCANNING, see *Nuclear Scanning*; *Ultrasound*

SCARLET FEVER, see *Skin Reaction*

SCHICK, see *Skin Reaction*

SCHILLER

In gynecological examinations, many doctors "paint" the cervix (entrance to the uterus) with an iodine solution in order to isolate any suspected area of disease. Normal cells contain glycogen (starch), which iodine will stain. Although the Schiller test is not a specific diagnostic tool, it does point out suspicious areas for further study. Before the cervix is stained, the cervical mucus (discharge) is also examined for threadiness (called spinnbarkeit). The time it takes for the thready components of the mucus to be stretched indicates the phase of the menstrual cycle (see **Tackmeter**).

When performed: During a routine gynecological examination; whenever the patient has a persistent vaginal discharge or bleeding or a vaginal infection that is not easily cured.

Normal values: After being painted with iodine, the cervix should show a uniform brown (sometimes slightly bluish brown) color.

Abnormal values: Any area of the cervix that does not take the stain and remains white or pink indicates a lack of normal starch-containing cells (most commonly from infection, cancer, or injury) and a bit of the unstained tissue should then be taken for **Biopsy**. False positive tests (lack of staining without subsequent disease) occur in one out of three patients.

SCHILLING (Vitamin B$_{12}$)

Vitamin B$_{12}$ (cobalamin) is essential to several bodily functions (tissue growth, nervous system functioning, and red blood cell production). Anemia is sometimes caused by a deficiency of vitamin B$_{12}$ in the diet, but the more common cause is a difficulty in absorbing vitamin B_{12} through the intestine. In pernicious anemia, the "intrinsic factor" (a protein in gastric secretion) does not join with the vitamin B_{12} ingested in the diet; as a result, the vitamin cannot be absorbed through the intestine into the blood.

In the Schilling test, the patient fasts for 8 to 12 hours and is then given radioactive vitamin B_{12} (cyanocobalamin) orally, followed by an intramuscular injection of nonradioactive vitamin B_{12} in sufficient amount to saturate the body with the vitamin. The amount of radioactive B_{12} that is absorbed and excreted is measured. All the urine over a 24-hour period is collected. Vitamin B_{12}, the "intrinsic factor," and antibodies to the "intrinsic factor" can also be measured directly from blood serum. These tests, although more accurate, are very expensive.

When performed: When the patient has symptoms of weakness and pallor; to aid in the diagnosis of certain anemias; following gastrectomy (surgical removal of the stomach).

Normal values: The total amount of radioactive vitamin B_{12} excreted in the urine is compared with the amount that was given to the patient. It should be from 8% to 40%, depending on the original amount administered and particular laboratory methods.

Abnormal values: Values between 2% and 8% are considered borderline. Values of less than 2% are seen in malabsorption of vitamin B_{12}, which can cause pernicious anemia and other megaloblastic anemias (oversized, immature red blood cells). Deficiency of vitamin B_{12} follows gastrectomy. It is also seen with alcoholism and intestinal infections, in people on certain vegetarian diets, in patients taking oral contraceptives or anticonvulsants, and in old age.

SCHIOTZ, see *Tonometry*

SCHIRMER'S

Schirmer's test measures whether the eye produces enough tears to keep it sufficiently moist. Usually a drop of anesthetic is placed in the eye and then a thin strip of filter paper is placed in the conjunctival sac (just inside the lower lid). The eyes are kept closed for five minutes; the paper is then removed and examined for tears (moisture). Tears normally come from lacrimal glands located in the upper outer corner of the eye and occasionally from the upper inner area. They empty into a tiny duct at the innermost corner of the eye and drain into the nose area.

Fluorescein Eye Stain is sometimes used to measure tearing; the fluorescein dye should disappear into the nasal duct within two minutes and be seen in the nasal cavity.

When performed: Whenever a patient complains of "dry eye" (most often when wearing contact lenses); whenever the eye waters constantly.

Normal values: The filter paper resting inside the eyelid should show almost half an inch of moisture after five minutes.

Abnormal values: The filter paper fails to show sufficient moisture with certain eye infections (such as conjunctivitis), vitamin A deficiency, and Sjögren's syndrome (an unexplainable disease found mostly in women past the menopause and usually associated with a very dry mouth and arthritis). Failure of tears to leave the eye can come from infection and blockage of the nasolacrimal duct (this condition may also be congenital and is easily treated by dilating the tear duct with a thin metal probe).

SCHISTOSOMIASIS, see *Agglutination*

SCHWABACH, see *Tuning Fork*

SCINTOGRAPHY, see *Nuclear Scanning*

SCOTCH TAPE, see *Feces Examination*

SCOTOMA, see *Visual Field*

SCREENING URINE EXAMINATION, see *Urine Examination*

SEDIMENTATION RATE (ESR)

The erythrocyte sedimentation rate (ESR), called "sed rate" by most physicians, is a measure in millimeters (mm) of how far the red blood cells (erythrocytes) cling together, fall, and settle toward the bottom of a specially marked test tube in an hour's time. The cells group together and then form a sediment, as mud does in still water. Essentially it is an indication of any infectious process going on in the body. The various methods of performing the ESR are labeled according to the different sizes and shapes of tubes (Cutler, Westergren, Wintrobe) in which whole blood, usually taken from a vein, is placed.

When performed: With any suspected infection or tissue damage; to detect if an unsuspected disease is present; to follow the progress of disease (an increased ESR that begins to return to normal is a good prognostic sign).

Normal values: Normal values differ slightly depending on the tube used: Cutler, 2 to 10 mm fall in one hour; Wintrobe, 0 to 20 mm fall in one hour; Westergren, 1 to 12 mm fall in one hour. In general, a fall of up to 10 mm in one hour in men is considered normal; in women and elderly people, rates of up to 20 mm in one hour are still within normal range.

Abnormal values: The ESR is increased (falls faster) with certain infections (not with typhoid fever or with most virus diseases), tissue damage as with heart attack (not with angina), rheumatic fever, rheumatoid arthritis (not degenerative arthritis), kidney disease, thyroid disease, and some other hormone disorders, some cancers, and many connective tissue diseases or autoimmune conditions. It is also increased after poisoning, during menstruation, and in pregnancy.

SEIDEL, see *Tonometry*

SELENIUM

Selenium is a trace mineral (required by the body in very minute amounts) and is essential for heart and other muscle function; it acts as a coenzyme (necessary for certain enzyme activity). It also seems to act on, and with, vitamin E as a protective antioxidant (prevents cell destruction) in the body. Selenium is found particularly in onions, garlic, meats, eggs, seafood (especially shellfish), leafy green vegetables, and most grains; the amount varies with the amount of selenium in the soil. No more than 150 mcg of selenium is needed in the daily diet, and if 1,500 mcg or more are eaten on a regular basis, toxic symptoms may develop. Whole blood taken from a vein may be tested, but more often selenium is measured in the urine.

When performed: With hair loss or brittle fingernails; when there is unusual irritability that cannot be explained; with certain liver diseases; when amyotrophic lateral sclerosis (degeneration of part of the spinal cord, causing paralysis) is suspected; in people whose occupation requires contact with certain electronic equipment containing selenium.

Normal values: Selenium levels of up to 0.2 mg per liter of blood and 0.1 mg per liter of urine are considered normal.

Abnormal values: Decreased values are found in people with heart disease, in early aging, and in some cases of muscular dystrophy. Increased values are found in patients with liver disease, fatigue, irritability, and excessive, early hair loss. Markedly increased amounts have been found in patients with amyotrophic lateral sclerosis.

SEMEN

The semen, seminal fluid, or ejaculate is the single most important test of testicle function and fertility. (Fertility has nothing to do with potency.) In barren marriages, 30% of the husbands are infertile; more than half of these men can be helped to become fertile. Beside sperm (spermatazoa), normal semen contains spermatocytes, Sertoli cells, sperm nutrients, red and white blood cells, macrophages, lecithin crystals, and secretions from the prostate as well as other glands (fructose, citric acid, proteins, prostaglandins, and hormones).

Semen is usually examined for volume, viscosity (thickness), **pH** (acidity), motility (movement: whether sluggish or quick), morphology (form and structure of sperm), amount of sperm (sperm count) and fructose level (deficient fructose levels in semen seem to parallel testicular hormone, or androgen, deficiency).

It takes approximately ten weeks for sperm to form, so that the sperm sample analyzed is actually indicative of bodily functioning over the preceding ten weeks. Thus a single examination that indicates irregularities cannot be considered valid. If any abnormality is noted, at least three more specimens should be examined for verification.

After sexual abstinence for four to six days, the patient collects a specimen either by masturbation or by coitus interruptus. Masturbation is preferable so that none of the sample is lost. Semen should be examined immediately, but no later than two hours after collection. The one exception is the postcoital (after-intercourse) test where, because of religious convictions or extreme embarrassment, the woman reports to her doctor as soon as possible after normal intercourse and the specimen is removed from the vagina.

When performed: As a test of gonadal function; in suspected infertility; after vasectomy to measure success of the surgery; when rape is suspected.

Normal values: Volume: the normal ejaculation is 2.5 to 5 ml of seminal fluid (about one teaspoon). A low-volume ejaculation (1 ml) may still be normal and may contain a high sperm count.

Viscosity: Semen seems to gel just after ejection but normally liquefies in 15 to 30 minutes. It should not be examined until it has liquefied.

pH: Normally the pH level ranges between 7.2 and 8.0 (slightly alkaline).

Motility: At least 70% to 90% of normal sperm are motile (active) in the first hour after ejection, and 50% should still be motile up to ten hours after ejection.

Morphology: In a sample, 80% to 90% of sperm should appear to have a normal form. The normal sperm has head, neck, and tail. Slight variations in the size and shape of the head (tiny, large, round, elongated and double heads) may be normal.

Sperm count: The normal semen sample contains 60 to 120 million sperm per ml. Patients who have more are not considered more fertile than others.

Fructose level: Normal fructose is 315 mg per 100 ml.

Abnormal values: Volume: A low volume of semen (less than 2.5 ml) may be, but is not always, associated with fertility problems unless accompanied by a low sperm count. An exceptionally high volume (more than 5 ml) can also be an indication of infertility.

Viscosity: Failure of the semen to liquefy from its gel form after 15 to 30 minutes may be associated with infertility.

Motility: Immobile or sluggish sperm are abnormal, and usually indicate infertility.

Morphology: Variation from the normal size and shape in more than 20% of sperm is indicative of infertility problems. The different ways the sperm takes up stain are significant. Frequency of senile or juvenile forms, diffuse staining, or lack of staining are abnormal variations. Usually the fewer the sperm, the more the abnormal forms that are seen.

Sperm count: A sperm count below 60 million per ml is considered abnormal. Organic disease of the genitals (mumps, prostatitis, occlusion of ducts), endocrine or other systemic disease, spinal cord injury, hypopituitarism, and even a form of anxiety (anorexia nervosa) can cause low or no sperm count.

Rape test: When there is a question of sexual intercourse, an examination for semen (especially sperm) may be performed. The presence and activity of sperm taken from the vagina may indicate the approximate time intercourse took place. If no sperm are found, suspected semen and/or vaginal fluid are sometimes examined for prostatic **Acid Phosphatase**, the presence of which usually indicates intercourse.

SEMINAL FLUID, see *Semen*

SENILITY, see *Cognitive Capacity Screening*

SENSITIVITY, see *Culture*

SENSORY

Many different tests measure a patient's ability to perceive various sensations (pain, a light touch, temperature differences, vibrations, etc.). Discovering the exact locations where sensations are decreased (or at times increased) can help indicate the area in the nerves or spinal cord where disease originates. In addition, when patients complain of unusual sensations (burning, tingling, pins and needles), tests must be performed to isolate the area involved.

In most sensory tests, the patient is asked to keep his eyes closed so that the sensitivity of the skin area being tested can be measured directly. Various objects (cotton, pins, tubes) are touched to or pressed on the skin to elicit a response. Sensory ability is affected by a great many conditions (injuries, tumors, drugs, poor nutrition, infection, and inherited diseases).

When performed: Whenever nerve, muscle, spinal cord, or brain disease is suspected; when patients complain of an inability to feel normal sensations or experience unusual sensations.

Normal values: A patient should be able to locate and discriminate between a pin prick on the skin, a touch with a piece of cotton, pressure from the doctor's hand, tubes containing warm and cold water applied to the skin, and a vibrating tuning fork touched to any bone area. The patient should be able to tell if a toe is being pushed up or bent down as well as which fingers and toes are being touched. These feelings should be equal on both sides of the body.

More discriminating types of sensory tests measure the ability of the brain to interpret sensation. For example, the skin may be touched at two points at the same time; normally a patient can describe the touching and how far apart the points are. Normal patients can also distinguish different materials that touch them (cotton versus silk), specific shapes, and letters or numbers that the doctor outlines with a finger on the palm of their hand or other skin area.

Abnormal values: Although any absence or diminution of sensory ability usually indicates disease, the area affected must always correspond to a specific nerve distribution, called a dermatome. For example, if the patient complains of loss of feeling in the knee area, a definite area above, below, and alongside the knee should also be affected. If the loss of feeling does not correspond to the anatomical distribution of the nerve, other causes for the complaint (hysteria, attempting to mislead the physician, etc.) must be considered.

SEROLOGICAL, see *Agglutination*; *Complement Fixation*

SEROTONIN

Serotonin (hydroxytryptamine) is manufactured in the blood from tryptophan (one of the amino acids in the protein we eat) and is then metabolized into 5-hydroxyindolacetic acid (HIAA), a compound that can be tested for in the urine. Serotonin acts to transmit nerve impulses and also constricts blood vessels. An excess of serotonin seems to be implicated in both flushing and blueness of the skin, rapid heartbeat, diarrhea, precipitation of asthma, and increased blood clotting (it is also found in the platelets). Exposure to the sun seems to increase serotonin production. Blood from a vein may be tested for serotonin, but testing of a 24-hour urine sample for HIAA is more common.

When performed: Primarily when a carcinoid tumor (usually in the intestinal tract) is suspected; when there is unexplained cyanosis (bluish color to the skin) and an enlarged liver.

Normal values: Serotonin in whole blood ranges from 0.05 to 0.20 mcg per ml. HIAA in urine ranges from 2 to 8 mg per 24-hour sample.

Abnormal values: With a carcinoid tumor (called an argentaffinoma), values of HIAA may go up to 1,000 mg per 24-hour urine specimen. Certain tranquilizers, antidepressant drugs, and foods that contain serotonin (such as avocados, bananas, pineapples, and eggplants) may cause elevated levels.

SERUM COMPLEMENT, see *Complement*

SERUM HEPATITIS (SH), see *Australian Antigen*

SERUM PROTEINS, see *Albumin/Globulin*

SEVENTEEN KETOSTEROIDS (17-KS), see *Cortisol*

SEX CHROMATIN, see *Chromatin*

SEX DETERMINATION, see *Amniocentesis*

SEXUAL IDENTITY, see *Chromatin*

SEXUAL POTENCY, see *Impotence*

SGOT, see *Glutamic Oxalacetic Transaminase*

SGPT, see *Glutamic Oxalacetic Transaminase*

SH, see *Australian Antigen*

SHINGLES, see *Herpes*

SHK-STI SYSTEM, see *Electrocardiogram*

SIA, see *Macroglobulin*

SICKLE CELL, see *Red Blood Cell*

SICKLE CELL HEMOGLOBIN (HEMOGLOBIN S), see *Hemoglobin*

SIGMOIDOSCOPY, see *Endoscopy*

SINUS CULTURE, see *Culture*

SJÖGREN'S SYNDROME, see *Schirmer's*

SKIN GRAFT, see *HL-A Antigen*

SKIN REACTION

Many diagnostic tests measure the allergic sensitivity of the skin as an indication of either susceptibility to or previous contact with disease-producing substances. Common skin reaction tests (also called intracutaneous, intradermal, or subcutaneous tests) include the tuberculin test and the purified protein derivative (PPD), which is similar to the tuberculin test; the Schick test for susceptibility to diphtheria; the Dick test for sensitivity to the Streptococcus toxin (scarlet fever); specific tests for tularemia, coccidioidomycosis, histoplasmosis, and trichinosis; and the various tests that measure allergic sensitivity to foods and pollens. Skin tests may also be used to detect immune reactions.

About 0.1 ml (much less than a drop) of the testing material is injected just under the top layer of the skin, producing a small, whitish bump. (If no bump is raised, the material has been injected too deeply.) The usual sites are the inner hairless portion of the lower arm and the back, but the injection can be made anywhere on the body. If the testing substance is mixed in a solution that in itself could cause an allergy, the mixing solution alone—without the testing element—is injected in the opposite arm as a control measure. Sometimes a tiny bandage soaked in the testing solution is placed on the arm and covered with adhesive tape; this is called a patch test. The newest test for allergies is called the radioimmunosorbent assay test (see **RAST**).

It should be noted that the Food and Drug Administration considers a number of commonly performed skin tests to be ineffective—specifically, those to test for mumps, trichinosis, histoplasmosis, lymphogranuloma, diphtheria, and the "old tuberculin" test for tuberculosis (the PPD is accepted by the FDA). The federal government is trying to remove the substances used in these tests from the market.

When performed: When allergy is suspected; to diagnose certain specific infections; in dermatological conditions that are difficult to diagnose; to measure immunological sensitivity.

Normal values: There are really no normal values for skin tests since positive responses do not always indicate the presence of disease. For example, a person who was once exposed to tuberculosis but who has no infectious activity whatsoever may still have a positive skin reaction. A person who has had diphtheria may have lost his immunity and thus have a positive reaction. With allergy tests, it is not unusual for the skin to react positively to certain substances that have no direct effect on the nose or lungs and that therefore may not be causing allergic disease in other parts of the body.

Abnormal values: Since a positive test may not necessarily be abnormal, any positive reaction must be interpreted in light of a patient's medical history and physical findings. A reaction is positive when the site of the injected material turns red and/or a raised bump (wheal) at least ¼ inch in diameter can be felt. The reaction generally appears 24 to 72 hours after the injection but may last for several days.

SLIT LAMP, see *Fluorescein Eye Stain*

SMELL FUNCTION

Smell function, or olfactory perception, refers to the ability to distinguish different odors. Before smell function can be determined, nasal airway resistance must be measured—usually with a pneumotachometer, an instrument that electronically indicates how much forced pressure is required to allow air to pass through the nasal cavity as well as the volume of air passed per second. At first both sides of the nose are measured together; then each side is measured separately. If resistance is found, a decongestant drug is instilled to shrink the nasal membranes and the test is repeated.

Once nasal resistance is eliminated, specific, familiar odors are introduced directly into one side of the nose and then the other. The Elsberg apparatus is used to ensure strict control of odor administration time. Tobacco, cloves, coffee, vanilla, and lemon are some characteristic odors used. (Other odors such as ammonia and menthol, while characteristic, should not be used because of their irritability; they will cause a "reaction" in the nose that the patient wrongly interprets as smell.) Smell function is usually tested along with **Taste Function**.

When performed: Whenever a patient complaints of the loss of aroma perception, especially the aroma of foods; whenever brain disease is suspected; following brain injury; in sinus infections; prior to rhinoplasty (plastic surgery of the nose) and to record the degree of deviation of the nasal septum in interfering with smell function.

Normal values: Most patients can perceive the smallest trace of a familiar odor when it is mixed with air and forced directly into the nose.

Abnormal values: Anosomia, or the total absence of smell, most commonly comes from brain tumors or injury to the nerve from the brain to the upper, inner portion of the nose. A loss of smell on only one side of the nose is even more suggestive of brain disease. People who have a disease of one particular area of the brain hallucinate smells but do not actually lose the sense of smell. Naturally, any condition (such as infection) that prevents odors from reaching the area of the nose that detects smell will also cause a false negative reaction (once the condition is cleared, normal smell returns).

SMOKING, see *Hemoglobin*

SNELLEN, see *Visual Acuity*

SODIUM

Sodium is one of the blood electrolytes. (Atoms or ions of **Bicarbonate**, **Chloride**, and **Potassium** are the other major electrolytes.) It is essential to maintaining the body's normal water metabolism and acid-base balance, and to keep the proper amount of fluids in the bloodstream and in the tissues *around* the cells (potassium holds the water *in* each cell). On a typical diet, the average adult takes in around 6 g (about 0.2 ounce) of sodium a day. The ingestion of excess sodium from salt (sodium chloride), monosodium glutamate (MSG), and the many heavily sodium-based flavor enhancers (such as disodium inosinate and disodium guanylate) found in processed foods can cause water retention (edema), headache, and several other symptoms. A loss of body sodium (from excessive sweating, vomiting, or fever) produces dehydration. Blood is taken from a vein and the serum is tested. Sodium is also measured in the urine, in sweat, occasionally in the spinal fluid, and in saliva.

When performed: When there is persistent water retention; to help diagnose various hormone disorders; to determine the cause of coma; to confirm suspected cystic fibrosis of the pancreas.

Normal values: Normal sodium levels range from 135 to 150 mEq per liter in serum and 40 to 200 mEq per liter in a 24-hour urine sample.

Abnormal values: Increased sodium levels (hypernatremia) are found in some endocrine disorders, especially those of the adrenal glands (Addison's disease); in dehydration; and in patients taking certain hormones and drugs such as steroids, contraceptive pills, and sodium-formulated medicines. Kidney disease, heart disease, and high blood pressure can also cause increased amounts of sodium in the blood. Decreased serum sodium is found in diabetes, inadequate adrenal function, and patients taking diuretic drugs.

Urine sodium usually parallels serum sodium, except with dehydration or with certain hormones or drugs that cause the kidney to excrete excessive amounts in the urine.

Sodium is greatly increased in sweat and in saliva (as are chlorides) with cystic fibrosis of the pancreas (mucoviscidosis), a congenital condition that usually expresses itself through repeated lung infections.

SOMATOTROPIN, see *Growth Hormone*

SONOGRAPHY, see *Ultrasound*

SOUND, see *Hearing Function*

SOUND CARDIOGRAM, see *Phonocardiogram*

SOUND SCANNING, see *Ultrasound*

SPATIAL ELECTROCARDIOGRAPHY, see *Vectocardiogram*

SPECIFIC GRAVITY (URINE), see *Mosenthal; Urine Examination*

SPEECH, see *Language Function*

SPERM, see *Semen*

SPINAL FLUID, see *Cerebrospinal Fluid*

SPINAL FLUID CULTURE, see *Culture*

SPINAL FLUID SCAN, see *Nuclear Scanning*

SPINNBARKEIT, see *Schiller*

SPIROMETRY, see *Pulmonary Function*

SPLEEN SCAN, see *Nuclear Scanning*

SPODICK-HAFFTY-KOTILAINEN: SYSTOLIC TIME INTERVALS, see *Electrocardiogram*

SPOT, see *Mononucleosis*

SPUTUM

Sputum is the mucous secretion (phlegm) from the lower respiratory system (the lungs, the bronchi, the trachea, and the larynx). The sputum examination usually does not include the nose or sinus secretions, which are part of the upper respiratory tract. In infections and other inflammatory conditions, sputum volume and viscosity (thickness) increase.

Sputum is collected for microbiologic **Culture** or **Cytology** examination. Some is placed on culture plates to check for bacterial growth, some is placed on slides for microscopic study, and some is examined by the Papanicolaou stain for tumor study. Most clinicians request a specimen of all the sputum a patient produces in a 24-hour period; a few find a single specimen sufficient for diagnostic study. Usually sputum is obtained by coughing. It can also be aspirated (suctioned) through a bronchoscope.

When performed: With suspected respiratory tract disease, when there is a persistent cough that cannot be explained, or with an undiagnosed general infection.

Normal values: Unless there is a disease process (infection, irritation, allergy, or cancer) very little sputum is produced. Any minute amounts of sputum produced should be clear, colorless, and odorless and should reveal no bacteria and very few cells or crystals under the microscope.

Abnormal values: An increased amount of yellow to greenish sputum indicates a lung infection. Reddish or brown sputum accompanies lung congestion with or without infection (pinkish, watery, foamy sputum is considered diagnostic of pulmonary edema).

In lung infections, there is a great increase in the white blood cells and fat crystals. With coliform bacteria and anaerobic infections, the sputum has an unpleasant odor. With allergy such as asthma, there is an increase in one particular white blood cell, the eosinophil, along with Curschmann's spirals and Charcot-Leyden crystals, which are quite different from the crystals seen in infection. With irritation (from dust, smog, etc.) an increase in the cells that line the bronchial passageways of the lung is seen. Elastic fibers found in the sputum on microscopic examination suggest a destructive process such as pneumonia, tuberculosis, cancer, or lung abscess.

SPUTUM CULTURE, see *Culture*

SQUINT, see *Strabismus*

STANDARD BICARBONATE, see *Bicarbonate*

STENGER, see *Tuning Fork*

STEREOPSIS, see *Visual Acuity*

STI, see *Systolic Time Intervals*

STOMACH CONTENTS, see *Gastric Analysis*

STOMACH HORMONE, see *Gastrin*

STOOL CULTURE, see *Culture*

STOOL EXAMINATION, see *Feces Examination*

STRABISMUS

Strabismus is a condition in which the two eyes do not see the identical image simultaneously; usually one eye is directed in a slightly different direction from the other. Most often this condition is the result of an eye muscle weakness (eye movement is controlled by six different muscles); it can also come from brain and nerve involvement. By having the patient look at fixed points in certain directions, the physician can determine the specific external ocular muscle at fault. Forms of strabismus include heterotropia (squinting); esotropia (cross-eyes), where one or both eyes look inward; exotropia (walleyes), where one eye always looks outward; and diplopia (double vision).

Diplopia is detected when a red glass is placed over one eye and the patient, looking at a light with both eyes, sees both a red and a white dot. In the Worth four-dot test, a red glass is placed over one eye and a green glass over the other; the patient looks at a special light that shows one red, one white, and two green dots. Depending on what the patient sees, the doctor can determine which eye is affected and whether the two eyes can work together.

In the Wirt stereopsis test, polarized-lens glasses are used to ascertain the degree and possibility of fusion (the ability to use both eyes together for three-dimensional viewing). In the cover-uncover test, a patient looks at an object 20 feet away first with one eye covered and then with the cover removed. The Hirschberg test, similar in technique, is used on young children who do not easily cooperate; movement of corneal light reflex is noted. The Maddox rod test uses cylinders to measure eye deviations. All the tests help confirm the specific cause of strabismus and help determine prognosis. About one in 20 children have a form of strabismus.

When performed: Whenever patients have cross-eyes, walleyes, squinting, or double vision; following head or eye injury; with all cranial nerve diseases; in patients with diabetes or vascular diseases.

Normal values: When both eyes look at the identical spot or object, they should see it as one rather than two distinct spots or objects, without blurring (in this instance blurring would be due to double vision rather than loss of **Visual Acuity**). The patient should be able to control each of the six muscles of the eye so that they move in perfect harmony.

Abnormal values: Deviations are measured in units of prisms. With strabismus, a prism lens must be placed in front of the eye to correct muscular weakness or nerve defect. One prism diopter (diopter is a unit of measurement in ophthalmology) means that at a distance of one meter (a bit more than three feet) the eye sees an image one centimeter away from its true location. In the Worth four-dot test, a patient with double vision will see five dots instead of four; whether the extra dot is red or green determines which eye is affected. In the cover-uncover test, when the cover is removed the weak eye will suddenly move instead of focusing in the direction that the uncovered eye is looking.

STREPTOCOCCAL INFECTION, see *Antistreptolysin O Titer*

STRESS (NERVOUS), see *Electromyography*

STRESS CARDIOGRAM, see *Electrocardiogram*

STRESS-INDUCING CIRCUMSTANCE, see *Jenkins Activity Survey*

SUBCUTANEOUS, see *Skin Reaction*

SUCCINYLCHOLINE REACTION, see *Cholinesterase*

SUCROSE HEMOLYSIS, see *HAM*

SUGAR, see *Glucose*

SUGAR WATER, see *HAM*

SULFHEMOGLOBIN, see *Hemoglobin*

SULKOWITCH, see *Calcium*

SUPERFICIAL REFLEX, see *Reflex*

SUPERFICIAL TACTILE SENSATION, see *Sensory*

SWEAT

Testing for the chemicals in sweat (see **Sodium**) helps to detect many different diseases. Measuring the ability to sweat is a particular test for physical as well as mental disease. A very weak iodine solution (in alcohol) is painted on the skin area under study and allowed to dry; the area is dusted with starch powder. The patient is then made to sweat (by administration of direct heat, hot liquids, or certain drugs). If the sweat glands are functioning properly, the white starch powder will turn dark blue.

When performed: Most often the test is performed to ascertain excessive sweating such as with "night sweats" (which occur only during sleep and suggest chronic infections); to differentiate malnutrition from certain specific diseases such as lupus erythematosus; to measure a spontaneous sweating reaction to anxiety.

Normal values: It is normal for sweat glands to function when exposed to direct heat, exercise, or excessive alcohol, or when the body is excessively warmed by clothes or blankets. Sweat may have a color if the body is exposed to certain chemicals (as in certain occupations) or if the sweat is accompanied by color-producing bacteria. Excessive bacteria can normally cause bromidrosis, or unpleasantly scented sweat, but this is usually limited to areas with skin folds.

Abnormal values: Hyperhidrosis, or excessive sweating under inappropriate conditions (as in a cool room), may be caused by vitamin deficiencies, hyperthyroidism, brain and spinal cord disease, blood vessel disease, and following surgery where certain nerves have been severed. Psychological problems usually cause excessive sweating on the palms of the hands and the soles of the feet. The inability to sweat is usually an inherited condition.

Note: The most recent type of sweat test involves taping and sealing a small piece of salt-treated blotting paper against the leg. After eight days, the amount of alcohol and/or acetaldehyde is measured. Patients who drink alcohol but deny it can be detected in this manner; patients with arrested alcoholism will have a negative sweat alcohol test.

SYMMETRIC TONIC NECK REFLEX, see *Reflex*

SYMONDS PICTURE STORY, see *Thematic Apperception*

SYNOVIAL FLUID

All body joints contain a small amount of straw-colored syrupy liquid called synovial fluid that helps lubricate the bone or cartilage surfaces. Three dozen different tests can be performed on joint fluid. The usual examination consists of measuring sugar levels and white blood cells, as well as searching for crystals, immunoglobulins, antigamma globulins, various forms of complement, and lupus erythematosus cells (see **Antinuclear Antibodies**). In the ropes test, the fluid is mixed with a mild acid to see if it forms a good mucin clot (a small, ropy-looking mass that stays together even with shaking).

In most instances, the patient is asked to fast the night before and the morning of the test so as not to abnormally alter the sugar level. The synovial fluid is obtained by inserting a small needle into the joint cavity (a process called arthrocentesis). Absolute sterile precautions must be observed to make sure that infection is not introduced into the cavity when the fluid is withdrawn. A joint cavity can contain up to half an ounce of fluid, but only one drop is needed to arrive at certain diagnoses.

When performed: Primarily when there is a swollen joint, whether hot and inflamed or not; to differentiate the different types of arthritis (from infectious to traumatic); to aid in the diagnosis of systemic lupus erythematosus; to follow the progress of any joint disease; when certain bleeding disorders are suspected.

Normal values: Normal synovial fluid is slightly yellow and clear with very few white blood cells (less than 200 per ml), no crystals, and a good mucin clot. Sugar levels and other chemical test values should approximate those found in normal plasma.

Abnormal values: With arthritis, synovial fluid tends to become more yellow or yellowish green and turns somewhat cloudy. The white blood cells increase markedly (over 10,000 per ml), and with certain diseases various types of crystals appear: uric acid crystals with gout, calcium crystals with pseudo-gout. With arthritis, the mucin clot is "poor"—that is, fragile and easily breakable on shaking; with gout, it is even more fragile. With infectious arthritis, synovial fluid sugar levels are reduced and the fluid is given a **Culture** test.

Note: A new test, the limulus assay (limulus is a special chemical), is now being performed whenever synovial fluid is suspected of being infected with Gram-negative bacteria (see **Gram Stain**); it can give a fairly reliable indication of infection within an hour as opposed to the several days needed to culture bacteria. The limulus test can also be used on blood to indicate the presence of small amounts of endotoxin (poisons from certain bacteria that can cause blood poisoning, sometimes called toxemia or sepsis).

THE ENCYCLOPEDIA OF

SYPHILIS

Many tests help to determine if syphilis is present in the body. These tests may be of the treponemal variety (looking for Treponema pallidum, the corkscrew-shaped organisms that cause the disease) or the nontreponemal variety of serological (blood) tests (see **Agglutination**; **Complement Fixation**) that give passive evidence of the disease if antibodies are present. The nontreponemal antigen tests include the Hinton, Kolner, Kahn, Kline, Mazzini, Wassermann, rapid plasma reagin (RPR), automated reagin (ART) and Venereal Disease Research Laboratory (VDRL). The VDRL is the most common test, but it is not completely accurate: one patient out of four with early syphilis will have a false negative reaction. These tests are not as expensive and are more easily performed than the treponemal tests, but they all may give false positive results in conditions other than syphilis (lupus erythematosus, malaria, leprosy, acute infections, and after smallpox vaccination).

The treponemal organisms are so narrow that they cannot be seen by ordinary microscopic light and need a "darkfield"; that is, they must be illuminated by reflected light in order to be observed. The darkfield examination is performed during the primary stage of syphilis; fluid from the lesion is placed on a glass slide and examined under the microscope for direct, living evidence of Treponema pallidum.

The Treponema pallidum immobilization test (TPI) takes serum from a suspected syphilis patient and adds it to complement (special serum antibodies); when both are then added to a virulent strain of live Treponema pallidum, the organisms become immobilized.

The Fluorescent Treponemal Antibody Absorption (FTA-ABS) test has been found to be more sensitive for syphilis than the TPI. It is easier to perform and therefore used more often, but one patient out of ten with very early syphilis will still be missed (have a false negative reaction). False positive reactions may occur when the patient's serum contains antinuclear factor, rheumatoid factor, or increased globulins. Blood from a vein is tested. Spinal fluid is also tested to detect latent syphilis and to follow the progress of treatment.

When performed: Whenever there is a mystifying infection (syphilis is known as the great masquerader, since it imitates many illnesses); when a skin disease does not heal; with other symptoms that cause suspicion of syphilis; when certain tropical diseases are suspected; when pregnancy is diagnosed.

In most states (with the exception of Maryland, Minnesota, Nevada, and South Carolina) a syphilis test is required by law before obtaining a marriage license.

Normal values: Normally there is no evidence (reaction) of syphilis in the body.

Abnormal values: The test is positive when there is active or even inactive (old) syphilis. Other conditions that can cause a positive reaction include malaria, Hansen's disease, rat-bite fever, pellagra, infectious mononucleosis, pneumonia, tuberculosis, and lupus erythematosus.

SYSTEMIC HYPERTENSION, see *Blood Pressure*

SYSTEMIC LUPUS ERYTHEMATOSUS, see *Antinuclear Antibodies*

SYSTOLIC PRESSURE, see *Blood Pressure*

SYSTOLIC TIME INTERVALS (STI)

The word "systole" refers to the time during which the heart contracts and pumps blood into the aorta and the rest of the vascular system ("diastole" is the time the heart relaxes between contractions). An electronic instrument is placed on the side of the neck so that the carotid artery pulse can be felt. The device records the pulse waves (pressure from the heart's contraction and forcible outflow of blood) in the form of specific waves that can be measured and timed.

Many cardiologists consider the STI to be the most accurate of all tests of heart muscle and vascular system functioning. It is usually performed along with a standard **Electrocardiogram** (ECG) and a **Phonocardiogram** (PCG). The first part of the STI measures the left ventricular ejection time, or how long it takes the left side of the heart to empty itself. The second part of the test measures the pre-ejection period (PEP), or the exact time the heart muscle is activated to the time the blood begins to leave the heart. The two parts of the STI can reveal heart disease that is not detected by other tests.

The most recent innovation for measuring systolic time intervals is the Spodick-Haffty-Kotilainen ear pulse wave recording (performed as a part of the 24-hour Holter-type **Electrocardiogram**).

When performed: When suspected heart disease patients have a normal stress electrocardiogram; to check the effectiveness of certain drugs on the heart as well as to uncover toxic effects of other drugs; to follow the progress of patients who have heart attacks.

Normal values: The left side of the heart should empty completely in less than 0.35 seconds, the pre-ejection period is even less.

Abnormal values: Prolonged systolic time intervals are seen with heart valve disease, with damaged heart muscle (usually after a heart attack), and with heart damage caused by certain cancer-treating drugs.

T3/T4, see *Thyroid Function*

TACKMETER

The tackmeter (tackiness viscometer) measures the cohesiveness or stickiness of the mucous secretion of the cervix by noting how much strength it takes to pull it apart. It is a particular test for ovulation time—that is, the exact moment when the ovary releases an egg ready for pregnancy. (Ovulation time is also measured by the **Body Temperature** test.) A version of this test can be performed by women at home.

When performed: To determine if a woman is fertile and does, in fact, ovulate or produce fertilizable eggs; after a woman stops taking birth control pills (to learn when she can become pregnant); as a means of birth control (to inform a woman of her "safe" days).

Normal values: Cervical mucus becomes thinner (less viscous) at the time of ovulation and thickens both before and afterward. Patients using the mucus examination as a means of birth control need to know only the difference between thick and thin; an expert in the field can evaluate the degree of viscosity accurately enough to predict ovulation time within a few hours.

Abnormal values: Failure of the cervical mucus to thin out during the menstrual cycle usually indicates failure to ovulate.

TANGENT SCREEN, see *Visual Field*

T-ANTIGEN

T-antigen, named after Dr. Oluf Thomsun of Denmark who discovered it, is a substance found on red blood cells that reacts with antibodies in patients who have the most common types of breast cancer. A tiny amount of T-antigen is injected into the skin, usually in the forearm, and the site of injection is examined again in 24 hours. The test seems to be able to detect breast cancer even before a tumor large enough for a **Biopsy** is formed.

When performed: When there is suspicion of breast cancer, and to help differentiate non-cancerous breast lumps from cancerous ones. The test is also being used experimentally for the early detection of other cancers.

Normal values: No skin reaction 24 hours after injection of T-antigen.

Abnormal values: An indurated (hard) reddish area at the site of the injection after a 24-hour period.

TARTRAZINE SENSITIVITY

Urticaria (hives), sinus problems, and asthma can be caused by reactions to different foods, drugs, and plants. A common cause of these symptoms is sensitivity to tartrazine, a substance that is found naturally in foods such as sweet potatoes and that is often added to foods as a coloring (Yellow Dye No. 5). Tartrazine is commonly used as a coloring in ice cream, candy, desserts, commercial pastries, certain vegetable oils, and butter. For many of these foods, federal law does not require that the coloring be listed among the ingredients; state laws require only an indication that coloring has been added (the specific name of the color need not be mentioned).

Most people who are sensitive to tartrazine are also allergic to aspirin and show this allergy by the same symptoms. Since it can be dangerous to test for aspirin allergy directly, the tartrazine test is used. The patient eats a tartrazine-free diet and takes no pills coated with the coloring for seven to ten days. If the usual allergic symptoms go away, the patient is given a specific dose of tartrazine; if sensitivity exists, the allergy will return within three hours.

When performed: Whenever a patient has repeated episodes of urticaria, asthma, or sinus allergies.

Normal values: There should be no skin or respiratory passage reaction to a large dose of tartrazine.

Abnormal values: A positive skin or respiratory reaction to a dose of tartrazine usually means the patient is also allergic to aspirin and products that contain or act like aspirin (certain drugs for arthritis and sodium benzoate, a food preservative).

TASTE FUNCTION

The ability to taste four distinctive flavors on both sides of the tongue equally is important to the diagnosis of certain brain lesions. Nerves of taste located on the front of the tongue come from a different part of the brain than nerves of taste located on the back of the tongue. Standardized solutions of 5% glucose (sweet), 5% salt, 1% quinine (bitter), and 1% vinegar (sour) are placed directly on both sides of the tongue from the front to the back with a dropper. Usually **Smell Function** tests are performed at the same time. In the Franklinic test, a small electric current is applied to the tongue and should cause a sour taste. The

Circulation Time test makes use of the ability to taste a bitter substance.

When performed: When brain disease is suspected; following brain or neck injury; with severe tooth problems; with liver, lung, heart, and stomach disease.

Normal values: All four standard flavors should easily be detected. The sweet taste is predominant at the tip of the tongue; the bitter taste, on the back surface. Sour tastes are detected along the sides, and salty flavors are picked up all over the front half of the tongue as well as along the sides.

Abnormal values: The most common cause of taste loss is Bell's palsy (paralysis of one of the main nerves to the face). Total loss of taste (ageusia) can also be the result of a brain or nerve tumor. It may occur, temporarily, with migraine attacks and in lung and liver disease. Hallucinations of taste, but not loss, can come from brain lesions and tongue infections, and during pregnancy.

TAT, see *Thematic Apperception*

TAY-SACHS, see *Amniocentesis*

TBG, see *Thyroid Function*

TEAL, see *Tuning Fork*

TEAR, see *Schirmer's*

TEMPERATURE, see *Body Temperature*

TENSILON

Tensilon is a brand name for edrophonium, a chemical that works at the nerve ends to stimulate muscle contraction. Because it works so rapidly but lasts for such a short period of time, Tensilon is used for the diagnosis of myasthenia gravis (a condition where the muscles, particularly of the face and neck, tire very quickly to the point of paralysis). It is given as an intravenous injection. Because of the possibility, though rare, that injection of edrophonium will cause nausea, diarrhea, excessive salivation, excessive sweating, and a slowing of the heart rate, atropine is kept ready to use as an antidote. (Edrophonium's action on the heart allows it to be used on occasion to stop attacks of extremely rapid heartbeat.) The drug should be administered with extreme caution in patients with asthma. Just before Tensilon is given, a placebo (an innocuous substance) is injected to make sure that the patient is not simply reacting to the test procedure itself. If there is no reaction to injection of the drug, a second dose may be given two to three minutes later (a few myasthenia gravis patients need a greater amount of the drug to be effective).

When performed: Primarily as a diagnostic test for myasthenia gravis; as an indication of overdose of one of the usual medications prescribed to treat myasthenia gravis.

Normal values: In a patient with weakened muscle strength or muscle paralysis (most commonly seen in the eyelids, which cannot be held open), muscle strength returns within one minute after injection of Tensilon, and the ability to use the muscles lasts for five to ten minutes.

Abnormal values: Weakened or paralytic muscles that respond to one or two injections of the drug indicate myasthenia gravis. On rare occasions, a patient with amyotrophic lateral sclerosis (muscle atrophy) will respond to Tensilon, but will not benefit from the usual myasthenia gravis treatment (drugs similar to Tensilon, but much longer-acting).

TERMAN, see *Intelligence Quotient*

TESTIS FUNCTION

There are several different tests to determine if the testicles (male gonads) are functioning normally (see **Chromatin**; **Semen**). Two tests in particular indicate whether the testes are performing their two basic functions: producing the male hormone testosterone and producing sperm. One is the direct measurement of testosterone in blood plasma or in the urine; the other is measurement of gonadotropin (chorionic gonadotropin) in both the blood and the urine.

Testosterone is also manufactured in small amounts in the liver and by the adrenal glands (women normally produce a very small amount of testosterone in their ovaries and adrenals). Thus testosterone testing is not an absolute measurement of testicle function; however, it is a reasonable approximation. Testosterone is the hormone responsible for secondary sex characteristics such as hair distribution, voice pitch, hip configuration, and muscle development (primary sex characteristics are the sex organs themselves).

In the past, the 17-ketosteroid (17-KS) test was used to evaluate testis function. It has since been learned that almost all 17 ketosteroids come from the adrenal glands and not the testicles, as was once believed; thus the test is no longer a measure of male organ activity.

Human chorionic gonadotropin (HCG) measurements in the urine seem to be the most significant indicator of testicular activity. Gonadotropin measured in blood taken from a vein is a confirmatory test. The measurement of human chorionic gonadotropin is also used to determine if a woman is pregnant (see **Pregnancy**).

When performed: Whenever a tumor of the reproductive glands (testis or ovaries), adrenal glands, pituitary gland, or hypothalamus is suspected; whenever congenital (inherited) sex defects are being considered; with hypogonadism (testicles that do not function adequately or failure of the testicles to descend), a condition that is usually not detectable until after puberty and at times until 21 years of age; with suspected prostate trouble; with impotence; as a possible indication of heart disease.

Normal values: Serum or plasma testosterone averages from 500 to 1,200 ng per 100 ml in men and from 25 to 50 ng per 100 ml in women. Men usually excrete up to 200 mcg in the urine every 24 hours; women and children excrete no more than 10 mcg per 24 hours. There should be no measurable gonadotropins in the blood or urine of men or women (except during pregnancy). At times, a 24-hour specimen of urine may contain from 5 to 50 mouse-uterine units of pituitary gonadotropins. (The test is measured by an increase in the weight of the mouse uterus after the mouse has been injected with the human specimen; pituitary gonadotropins are slightly different from chorionic gonadotropins).

Abnormal values: Testosterone levels are decreased in hypogonadism and indicate inadequate or absent testis function such as can be caused by alcohol and many other drugs. Urine and blood pituitary gonadotropin levels are increased when hypogonadism originates in the testicle rather than the pituitary gland or hypothalamus. They are usually decreased when hypogonadism is caused by pituitary problems. Chorionic gonadotropins are increased with testicular tumors. Low testosterone levels, only in conjunction with elevated estradiol (female hormone) levels, have been implicated in susceptibility to heart disease (see **Estrogen**).

TESTOSTERONE, see *Testis Function*

THALLIUM SCAN, see *Nuclear Scanning*

THEMATIC APPERCEPTION (TAT)

The thematic apperception test is a projective (information-provoking) technique in which the subject projects or reads into a series of pictures his own feelings and interpretations. The test was developed by the psychologist H. A. Murray in 1938. It is based on the hypothesis that an individual will view each of the pictures in the light of his own experience, and that the themes of the stories the individual tells about each picture will reveal much about his social and emotional adjustment as well as his attitudes toward sex, authority, and aggression.

The examiner shows the subject one picture at a time and asks him to tell a complete story about the picture, the characters in the picture, how they feel, and what the outcome will be. The examiner records the stories and then discusses them with the subject. Later he makes interpretations from the material developed.

Scoring techniques are based on a number of criteria: whether the subject uses the whole picture or only part of it to develop his story; the characters and emotional tone of the story; and the type of ending. Interpretation of the data is usually based less on the formal scoring than on the interpreter's previous experience with personality patterns that have been suggested by the themes of the stories. As with other projective tests, there is always the danger of the examiner making arbitrary judgments that conform to his personal experience and beliefs. The examiner, therefore, will often tend to validate preconceived notions through such tests.

A number of variations on the TAT have been developed for specific purposes, such as evaluating handicapped children or ethnic groups and for vocational counseling. The children's apperception test (CAT) uses pictures of animals in social situations in the belief that young children will respond more readily to animals. The CAT-H, a version for older children, uses human figures in the same social situations as the animals in the CAT. The Bellak TAT uses the CAT pictures with a different concept of interpretation.

The Symonds Picture Story uses pictures especially oriented to adolescents.

The Blacky Pictures have a psychoanalytic or Freudian orientation. The child is shown pictures of a dog named Blacky and his family and is encouraged to tell the therapist about his own family and relate the pictures to them. Proponents of this test believe that it demonstrates the validity of psychoanalytic concepts. The Make-a-Picture Story (MAPS) uses a miniature empty stage (with various settings to choose from, such as bedrooms and bathrooms). The subject is offered mounted, cut-out figures (young, old, nude, animals, etc.) to place on the stage and explain why the particular figures were chosen and who and what they represent.

When performed: The TAT is used with normal subjects to study thinking processes, family relationships, attitudes toward sex and authority, cultural differences in minority and ethnic groups, and general levels of intelligence. It is also performed when there is suspicion of neurosis or other mental problems, as a measure of the emotional component of some physical illnesses (asthma, ulcers, headache) and as an indicator of progress during psychotherapy.

Normal values: Normal responses are generally those given most commonly by subjects. The test may furnish leads about the individual that the individual would find difficult to express in other ways.

Abnormal values: There is an assumption that evidence of emotional conflict, depression, aggression, phobias, fears, suicidal tendencies, or homosexuality will be revealed by the subject's interpretations of the pictures.

THERMOGRAPHY

Thermography measures the slightest variations in temperature of soft tissue in the body using infrared heat sensors. The technique is often used in mammography (breast examination) to detect any growth in the breast (the mass will have a different temperature from other breast tissue). Thermography may also be used on an extremity, particularly the leg, to help diagnose a thrombus (clot) in a vein. The inflammation usually associated with the thrombus raises the temperature in the area of the clot. Measuring temperature changes of the penis, especially after showing a patient sexually stimulating illustrations, can help differentiate physical from psychological impotence. The area of the body to be tested is usually placed on a heat-detection device that reacts to specific temperatures, either by color changes or a direct display of temperatures.

When performed: To aid in diagnosing breast masses; when thrombus is suspected; when other vascular conditions exist such as arterial circulation deficiencies, either from a nerve problem or as a direct defect (blood clot); to ascertain skin and adjacent tissue status (as in instances of possible gangrene).

Normal values: There are no strict normal values except in relation to other tissue; temperature response should reflect the type of tissue and the blood supply of the tissue being tested.

Abnormal values: Any unexpected change in tissue temperature in relation to surrounding tissue is considered abnormal.

THIAMIN (Vitamin B₁)

Vitamin B₁ (thiamin or thiamine) deficiency occurs most commonly in people with alcoholism and whose diet consists mainly of polished rice. High-carbohydrate diets may also cause vitamin B_1 deficiency. Thiamin is found in large amounts in yeast, meats, eggs, whole grains, and beans. Because this vitamin is not stored in the body, it must be replenished daily.

Beriberi is a specific disease caused by vitamin B_1 deficiency. Symptoms include cardiovascular irregularities (palpitation with gallop rhythm, abnormal electrocardiogram, venous pressure elevation, shortness of breath, edema), emotional irritability, loss of memory, anxiety, sluggish gastrointestinal activity, weakness, loss of ankle-jerk and knee-jerk reflexes, and inflammation of peripheral nerves. Both urine and blood can be analyzed for thiamin levels. Red blood cell enzymes can also indicate thiamin levels.

When performed: Whenever there is nervous system disease—loss of sensations (touch) or muscle problems; with undiagnosed heart disease or unexplained edema (water retention).

Normal values: The normal range of thiamin in whole blood is 1.5 to 4 mcg per 100 ml. Normal urine levels range from 25 to 75 mcg per 100 ml.

Abnormal values: Lower than normal values in either blood or urine indicate vitamin B_1 deficiency. Vomiting and diarrhea can also cause temporary B_1 deficiency.

THORACENTESIS

Thoracentesis is the removal of fluid from the space around the lungs. Normally no fluid is present. When evidence of fluid is found, usually after **Radiography** (X-ray) or **Ultrasound** testing of the chest, a small needle is inserted between the ribs (the X-ray shows exactly where) and the liquid is removed for further study to isolate bacteria, to look for blood cells, to perform a **Cytology** test and to perform various chemical tests for enzymes, glucose, and proteins. Because coughing can cause difficulty, a cough-suppressant medicine is usually given to the patient just prior to the test. At times, thoracentesis is also performed to remove large amounts of fluid and thus make breathing easier. Afterward, another chest X-ray is taken to make sure the lung did not collapse as a result of the test.

Paracentesis is the removal of fluid from the peritoneal cavity (the sac in the abdomen that holds the intestines). Normally, an accumulation of fluid does not exist in the peritoneal cavity, but when it does (called ascites), it indicates disease. A needle is inserted through the abdominal wall and the fluid withdrawn. Studies similar to thoracentesis are performed; ascites usually results from cancer, liver disease, and infections.

When performed: Whenever a patient has breathing difficulties; when a chest X-ray shows fluid around the lungs; when chest infection, fungus, or cancer is suspected; with heart or kidney failure causing edema; in certain forms of arthritis and rheumatoid disease; in certain bleeding-tendency diseases.

Normal values: There should be no measurable amount of fluid in the lung area.

Abnormal values: Any amount of fluid, called an effusion, is abnormal. Very low glucose levels in pleural (lung) fluid indicate rheumatoid diseases. Increased white blood cells in the fluid are found with cancer and infections.

Increased **Lactic Dehydrogenase** (LDH) is almost always found with lung cancer. Increased **Amylase** suggests disease of the pancreas. Increased protein usually signifies an infectious or hemorrhagic process. Decreased protein usually indicates heart, kidney, or liver failure.

THROAT CULTURE, see *Culture*

THROMBOCYTE, see *Platelet Count*

THROMBOSIS, see *Plethysmography*

THYMOL TURBIDITY (Thymol Flocculation)

Thymol turbidity is a test of liver function. The patient should avoid fatty foods and fatty liquids (milk, ice cream sodas) for at least 12 hours before the test. Blood is collected from a vein and the serum is added to thymol, a phenol chemical from the oil of thyme; the degree of turbidity (cloudiness) is then measured. The **Cephalin Flocculation** test is usually performed along with thymol turbidity to discriminate between various liver diseases.

When performed: When there is suspicion of liver disease; to distinguish between the various causes of jaundice; to follow the progress of treatment for liver disease.

Normal values: Normally the serum exhibits less than 5 measurable units of turbidity.

Abnormal values: Thymol turbidity is increased in certain liver diseases such as hepatitis (it may be normal in cirrhosis).

THYROID FUNCTION

There are a great many ways to assess how the thyroid gland is functioning. The primary tests consist of measuring the amounts of triiodothyronine (T_3) and thyroxine (T_4), both of which comprise the thyroid hormone. The hormone is made by the thyroid gland from tyrosine (an amino acid from protein) and iodine (which can enter the body through the skin and lungs as well as by diet). T_3 is four times as powerful as T_4, and only about half as much T_3 as T_4 is made each day. It is believed that T_3 is the "true" thyroid hormone, while T_4 may be a precursor of it.

Thyroid hormone is essential for normal growth and development, control of oxygen metabolism (energy), and production of other hormones such as the sex hormones and insulin. Thyroid hormone components are usually bound to serum proteins but unbound, or free T_4, is sometimes measured; free T_4 parallels T_4 except when certain drugs (oral contraceptives) are taken. T_3 and T_4 concentrations are measured directly in the serum. T_3 is also measured by its "uptake" (T_3U), which also shows how much thyroxine is already bound to serum proteins. Another commonly performed test of thyroid function is thyroxine-binding globulin (TBG), a measure of the major serum proteins to which T_3 and T_4 attach themselves. At least two different tests must be performed to understand the specific cause of thyroid disease so that appropriate treatment may be prescribed.

Other thyroid function tests that may be performed, usually when the tests described above are not conclusive, include the long-acting thyroid stimulator test (LATS), performed on babies whose mothers have thyroid disease, and various tests to detect thyroid autoantibodies (antithyroglobulin antibody, or ATA, and thyroid microsomal antibody, or TMA), which are produced when the thyroid gland acts as if it were infected and the body's immune protection system turns against itself in response. When cancer or nodules are suspected, a radioactive iodine screening test is performed.

In the thyroid stimulation test (TSH), the patient is given pituitary gland thyroid-stimulating hormone; by observing its effect on the thyroid, the physician can determine if thyroid problems are coming from the pituitary gland rather than the thyroid itself. An older test, rarely used today, is the protein-bound iodine (PBI), which essentially measures thyroxine (T_4) amounts (but not as accurately as the newer direct T_4 measurements). The simplest routine chemical confirmation test of thyroid function is **Cholesterol**.

The **Basal Metabolic Rate** (BMR), one of the first tests devised for thyroid function, is based on a different measurement principle from the usual thyroid function tests (oxygen consumption rather than measurement of chemicals in the blood). The BMR is used when the more sophisticated thyroid function tests cannot be performed (for example, when laboratory facilities are not available or when the patient has taken, or been in contact with, too much iodine to allow proper chemical measurement).

In the Achilles reflex (ankle-jerk) test, or photomotography, the heel tendon that moves the foot downward is struck with a rubber hammer. The force of the reflex activity of the foot and the time it takes the tendon to react are considered measures of thyroid gland activity.

The neonatal hypothyroidism test measures the amount of thyroid hormone in the newborn infant. Diagnosis of cretinism at birth allows treatment to prevent one form of mental retardation.

Blood is taken from a vein for the chemical tests and the serum is tested. Certain tests may be performed by using a drop of blood from the fingertip or earlobe. The tests can give false values if the patient has had any sort of iodine test in the six previous months (gall bladder X-rays, kidney X-rays; bronchograms, etc., using contrast dye) or has had excessive iodine in the diet for the previous month. Previous radioactive tracer tests can also cause erroneous results. Some thyroid function tests (PBI, radioactive iodine) may be performed on urine, saliva, and feces.

When performed: Whenever there is suspicion of a thyroid disorder; when other hormone disease is suspected; in all cases of depression; to follow the progress of treatment of thyroid disease; to screen newborn children for cretinism.

Normal values:
Free T_3: 100 to 250 ng per 100 ml
T_3U: 25% to 35%
T_4: 2.8 to 6.4 mcg per 100 ml
Free T_4: 3 to 5 ng per 100 ml

TBG: 10 to 26 mcg of T_4 per 100 ml

PBI: 3.5 to 8.5 mcg per 100 ml

LATS and thyroid antibodies are not normally present in the serum. Radioactive iodine uptake should range from 10% to 20% in the first hour and no more than 50% in 24 hours.

Abnormal values: Hyperthyroidism (Graves' disease, thyrotoxicosis, toxic goiter) usually shows increased T_3, T_4, radioactive iodine, and PBI, low cholesterol values, a normal amount of TBG, and low TSH (see **Exophthalmometer**). Hypothyroidism (goiter, cretinism, pituitary disorder) usually shows decreased T_3, T_4, radioactive iodine, and PBI, and high cholesterol values, an increased amount of TBG, and an elevated TSH. Thyroiditis (inflammation of the gland) may exist with hyperthyroidism or hypothyroidism, and the tests reflect the way the thyroid is (or is not) functioning. Tumors of the thyroid (cancers, cysts) may also alter the tests depending on how the growth affects function. Certain drugs such as estrogens and contraceptive pills will increase T_4, TBG, and PBI. Male hormones and other steroid drugs, as well as Dilantin, will cause low T_4, TBG, and PBI. While T_4 changes with some drug use, free T_4 stays normal. Pregnancy can cause false abnormal values such as elevated T_3, T_4, and TBG. Chronic kidney disease causes low T_3, T_4, and TBG along with an elevated T_3U. Excessive exposure to iodine increases PBI and decreases the radioactive iodine uptake. The taking of thyroid preparations usually increases all values. Large doses of aspirin, antiarthritic drugs, and anticoagulant drugs can alter thyroid function tests.

THYROID SCAN, see *Nuclear Scanning*

THYROXINE-BINDING GLOBULIN (TBG), see *Thyroid Function*

THYROXINE (T_4), see *Thyroid Function*

TICK FEVER, see *Complement Fixation*

TICKING WATCH, see *Hearing Function*

TIDAL VOLUME, see *Pulmonary Function*

TIMED VITAL CAPACITY, see *Pulmonary Function*

TOCOPHEROLS (Vitamin E)

Deficiency of vitamin E (really a group of related tocopherol oil compounds, with the alpha form the most active) is rare in the healthy adult who eats a normal diet. However, people who have increased their consumption of polyunsaturated oils (corn, safflower, cottonseed, or soybean) often are found to have vitamin E deficiency, which can cause the destruction of red blood cells. Vitamin E deficiency is known to cause anemia in infants and can cause infertility problems (inability to become pregnant). The vitamin does not have anything to do with sexual performance or potency, as has been erroneously reported. Vitamin E seems to help prevent tissue damage from smog. Blood is taken from a vein and the plasma is examined.

The erythrocyte (red blood cell) hemolysis test is an indirect, but easier to perform measure of vitamin E in the body. Red blood cells are destroyed in proportion to the lack of vitamin E.

When performed: When anemia is present; when smog is a severe lung irritant; when unexplained infertility exists; in malnutrition; when patients are on excessive polyunsaturated fatty acid diets.

Normal values: The tocopherol level is normally 0.5 mg per 100 ml of plasma.

Abnormal values: Less than 0.5 mg per 100 ml of plasma causes red blood cell destruction. Higher than normal values may also produce symptoms. People who take excessive amounts of vitamin E supplements have been reported to have swelling, particularly of the face and the breasts. Many plastic surgeons prohibit the taking of vitamin E supplements for a month prior to cosmetic surgery.

TOMOGRAPHY, see *Computerized Tomography*; *Radiography*

TONOMETRY

Tonometry is the specific measurement of the intraocular pressure (pressure of the fluid within the eyeball). It is used primarily to test for glaucoma, although there are rare instances of intraocular hypertension without glaucoma. Most glaucoma is of the chronic open-angle type, which does not occur until late in life and can usually be treated medically. The usual symptoms of glaucoma are poor vision (blurring), usually in only one eye at first, followed by gradual restriction of the **Visual Field**.

A Schiotz tonometer is placed on the pupil after a drop of anesthetic has been applied to the eye, and a gauge records the resistance of the eye to the slight pressure applied. The tonometer translates the resistance into millimeters (mm) of mercury (Hg). The procedure is similar to applying a contact lens to the eye. In another technique, called applanation, a drop of dye is placed on the eye and the slight pressure is applied and measured while the eye is observed through a special microscope. Tonometry should always be performed in a cool, dark room or false negative values will be recorded, missing the patient with glaucoma.

When the routine test result is equivocal, procedures to increase eye pressure are performed. In the water provocative test, the patient drinks a full quart of water at one time; the intraocular pressure is measured 30, 45, and 60 minutes later. If the pressure rises more than 8 mm Hg during that time, glaucoma is a reasonable diagnosis. In tonography, constant, gentle pressure is applied to the eye (using a special tonometer) for four minutes; the pressure should cause a decrease in the measured tension in normal individuals. If it does not decrease, glaucoma is the most likely diagnosis.

The Seidel test places the patient in a dark room for one hour. An increase in eye pressure during that time means that the ocular fluid does not escape when the pupils are dilated, as it normally should. A somewhat similar test is performed by dropping the drug homatropine into the eye. Homatropine causes the pupil to dilate. After an hour the eye is checked for any increase in pressure; an increase indicates glaucoma.

When performed: Tonometry is routinely performed on individuals over 40 years of age and on younger people whenever there is any vision difficulty (especially blurring) or any history of glaucoma in the family. It is also performed after any eye infection, after eye injury, with diabetes, and when there are thyroid problems.

Normal values: Normally the intraocular pressure measures between 10 and 20 mm Hg. Many physicians, through experience, can place fingers over the closed eye and the bony ridge above the eye and accurately detect normal intraocular pressure (less than 20 mm Hg).

Abnormal values: Lower than normal intraocular pressure (less than 10 mm/Hg) is rare and is usually due to an infection or sometimes follows surgery. A false lower value may occur in patients taking diuretics. Repeated pressure readings between 20 and 30 mm Hg (these readings must be taken several times; one or two tests are insufficient for diagnosis) indicate ocular hypertension and a presumption of glaucoma. Readings greater than 30 mm/Hg are almost always diagnostic of glaucoma, especially when accompanied by certain changes in visual field. Many drugs can cause increased intraocular pressure, which can then lead to glaucoma. Drugs that dilate the pupils, steroids, anticholinergics (such as used for bowel and bladder relaxation), antidepressants, antihistamines, muscle relaxants, and oral contraceptives are particularly dangerous, especially with patients who have a family history of glaucoma.

TOTAL BILIRUBIN, see *Bilirubin*

TOTAL CHOLESTEROL, see *Cholesterol*

TOTAL LIPIDS, see *Lipids*

TOTAL PROTEINS, see *Albumin/Globulin*

TOURNIQUET, see *Capillary Fragility*

TOURNIQUET TEST FOR VARICOSE VEINS

The varicose vein incompetency tests are performed to determine if leg varicosities are caused by diseases of the deep veins as opposed to problems of the superficial veins (which can be seen on the surface). The patient's leg is elevated to empty the veins, and a tourniquet is applied in various areas (above and below the knee, thigh, and calf). The patient stands (Trendelenberg test) and/or walks (Perthes test), and the leg is observed to ascertain how long it takes for the superficial veins to fill.

When performed: When varicose veins cause fatigue and discomfort; when there is lower-leg dermatitis or ulcer; to discover whether the varicosities are from some condition other than vein disease (such as pregnancy or abdominal tumor); when surgery is anticipated on the surface veins (to ascertain that after surgery the deep veins will be competent, or able to carry blood).

Normal values: When the deep veins are normal, the superficial veins fill 30 seconds after the leg is lowered (with the tourniquet still in place).

Abnormal values: If, when the leg is lowered and the veins fill immediately, the connecting veins between the deep and superficial systems are not adequate, surgery will be deemed to be of no help. If, while the tourniquet is on there is cramping or immediate filling while walking, there will probably be no benefit from surgery.

TOXEMIA OF PREGNANCY, see *Rollover*

TOXICOLOGY, see *Drug Monitoring*

TOXOPLASMOSIS, see *Agglutination*

TPI, see *Syphilis*

TRACER, see *Nuclear Scanning*

TRANQUILIZER, see *Barbiturates*

TRANSAMINASE, see *Glutamic Oxalacetic Transaminase*

TRANSAXIAL TOMOGRAPHY, see *Computerized Tomography*

TRANSFERRIN (IRON-BINDING CAPACITY), see *Iron*

TRANSFUSION, see *Typing and Cross-Matching*

TRANSHEPATIC CHOLANGIOGRAPHY, see *Radiography*

TREADMILL, see *Electrocardiogram*

TRENDELENBERG, see *Tourniquet Test for Varicose Veins*

TREPONEMAL PALLIDUM IMMOBILIZATION, see *Syphilis*

TRICHINOSIS, see *Agglutination*

TRIGLYCERIDE, see *Lipids*

TRIIODOTHYRONINE (T3), see *Thyroid Function*

TRUE CHOLINESTERASE, see *Cholinesterase*

TSH, see *Thyroid Function*

TUBAL PATENCY, see *Rubin*

TUBELESS GASTRIC ANALYSIS, see *Gastric Analysis*

TUBERCULIN, see *Skin Reaction*

TULAREMIA, see *Agglutination*

TUNING FORK

Tuning forks are metal instruments that vibrate when struck, giving off a pure tone of a predetermined number of cycles per second (cps). They are commonly used to tune pianos or other musical instruments. In medicine, tuning forks are used primarily to measure the ability to hear sounds by both air and bone conduction (see **Hearing Function**); they are also used to measure bone conduction sensitivity in other parts of the body as part of a neurological examination.

The base of the vibrating tuning fork is placed against a bone area (elbows, knees, ankles) and the sensation is noted by the patient as well as the equalness of the sensation on opposite sides of the body. There are five basic tuning-fork tests for hearing.

Weber: The base of the vibrating tuning fork is placed in the center of the forehead at the hairline, and the patient is asked if he hears the tone better in one ear than the other. Normally the tone is heard equally in both ears.

Rinné: The tuning fork is vibrated and placed next to each ear opening (for air conduction) and then against the mastoid bone behind the ear (for bone conduction) to see which tone is heard longer. Normally the tone will be heard much longer via air conduction (through the ear canal).

Schwabach: The physician vibrates the tuning fork and compares his perception of the tone with that of the patient. Assuming the doctor has normal hearing, the perceptions should be about the same.

Stenger: With the patient blindfolded, two tuning forks of the same tone are vibrated about an inch from each ear at the same time. The forks are then moved away from the ears. Normally the tone is heard in each ear from similar distances. If one ear is bad, the tuning fork will not be heard when it is placed close to that ear.

Teal: When a patient says he cannot hear the tuning fork via air conduction, the Weber test is again performed with the patient blindfolded. On the second trial, a nonvibrating fork is placed against the bone behind the ear and a second, vibrating fork is held a short distance away from that ear. If the patient is really deaf, he will not hear the tone; if he is simulating deafness, he will claim to hear the tone, although he is really hearing the second tuning fork.

Normal values: Each tuning fork test should be felt or heard equally on both sides of the body. Normal, or expected results for each hearing test are described above.

Abnormal values: Whenever the vibrations of a tuning fork are not felt or heard, or where one side of the body perceives the vibrations differently from the other side. Abnormal values for specific hearing tests are described above.

TYMPANOMETRY

Tympanometry is a test to measure the functioning of the eardrum. Under controlled pressures, tones of different frequency are applied to the external ear (the outer ear canal, which leads to the eardrum) and are monitored by a microphone as differences in pressure are administered. A small plug containing three tiny tubes is inserted into the ear canal and the pressure as a response to sound is recorded on a graph. The test is twice as effective as direct examination of the ear with an otoscope (looking into the ear) for detecting middle-ear infection (otitis media).

When performed: Primarily in infants and schoolchildren who are not prone to cooperate when being examined directly for otitis media; whenever there is suspicion of middle-ear infection in patients who will not allow direct examination, particularly when a patient has repeated ear infections; when aspiration of the middle-ear chamber (deliberately putting a hole in the eardrum to obtain material for diagnosis) is not possible; whenever allergy is suspected as a cause of ear problems.

Normal values: From 10 to 40 millimhos (mmho), depending on the frequency of the tone and pressure applied.

Abnormal values: No matter what the frequency of the tone, the detected mmho is usually reduced in half when there is middle-ear infection or fluid (usually pus) in the middle-ear chamber.

TYPE A/TYPE B PERSONALITY, see *Jenkins Activity Survey*

TYPHOID FEVER, see *Agglutination*

TYPHUS, see *Agglutination*

TYPING AND CROSS-MATCHING

Typing and cross-matching are performed to determine a person's blood type. Blood may be typed according to the common A, B, AB, and O groups (called the ABO system), the Rh positive and Rh negative groups (called the Rh system, which now has many additional subgroups), the MNS's system, or the Kell system. There are nearly 100 known blood group systems at present. Typing is essentially an **Agglutination** procedure to search for certain antibodies in the blood.

When a transfusion is prescribed by a doctor (usually after severe blood loss or during surgery), knowledge of the type of blood of both the donor and the recipient is not enough. Donor blood may be labeled as the same type as that of the patient, but the two must still be specifically cross-matched (mixed) to prevent an incompatible transfusion, which causes hemolysis (destruction of the red blood cells) and can be fatal. Most commonly the donor's red blood cells (which contain the antigens or agglutinating-precipitating factor) are tested for any possible reaction to the patient's serum (which contains the antibodies or response to agglutinating-precipitating factor). At times, the blood may also be tested for sickle cells prior to transfusion.

When performed: The test is performed whenever a blood transfusion is prescribed. A patient about to have surgery will often have his blood typed and cross-matched with potential donors well ahead of time.

Normal values: There should be no evidence of agglutination or hemolysis when the blood of the donor and the recipient are mixed.

Abnormal values: Any evidence of agglutination when the two different blood samples are mixed indicates incompatibility.

UCG, see *Pregnancy*

ULCER, see *Gastrin*

ULTRASOUND

Ultrasound is a diagnostic technique that uses sound waves to create a "picture" of certain areas of the body. The technique is similar to an X-ray, but without any of the dangers of radiation exposure; although the absolute safety of ultrasound is also being questioned. High-frequency sound waves (above the range of human hearing) are directed toward a body organ or cavity. The sound echoes back from the selected organ or tissue to form the "picture." The procedure is performed with a transducer (a microphonelike instrument that emits sounds and also detects the echo), which is touched to the body over the area to be studied. Before the transducer is used, a coating of mineral oil is applied to the skin to prevent any air from coming between the body and the instrument. The results may be reproduced in graphic form (resembling an electrocardiograph record) or as shadow illustrations; the latter are especially important for determining the exact location of the fetus during pregnancy (see **Amniocentesis**). The **Echocardiogram** also uses ultrasound as a measuring technique.

At times sound waves that are reflected back from moving objects (such as the heartbeat or blood flow through an artery or vein) show a change in frequency with changes in the speed of movement. This is called the "Doppler effect," and measurement is known as Doppler ultrasonography. Such tests are particularly valuable in discerning the heartbeat of the fetus and in measuring the arterial blood flow to and in the brain as a means of detecting and even preventing stroke.

In cases of suspected deep-vein thrombosis (see **Plethysmography**), the tests can sometimes ascertain whether blood is easily flowing through the vein or is blocked by a clot.

With recent developments in ultrasound techniques, the illustrations produced can, in many instances, achieve similar results to **Computerized Tomography** without the hazards of X-ray and at a lower cost. For example, ultrasound scanning can show up a mass in the abdomen (liver, gall bladder, spleen, pancreas, kidney); of even greater value, it can show if the mass is cystic (containing fluid, such as an abscess) or solid (tumor). Lesions only an inch in size can be detected by ultrasonography. An echoencephalogram (brain scan by ultrasound) can show if there are any tumors or other masses (clots or hemorrhages) in the brain. An eye sonogram can reveal pathology inside the eye when there is no other way of seeing inside (see **Fundoscopy**). The thyroid, prostate, and lymph glands may also be tested with ultrasound. An ultrasound scanner is portable and can be brought to the bedside of a patient too ill to move.

When performed: After head or abdominal injury; whenever a mass is suspected in the head or abdomen; whenever there is undiagnosed pain in the abdomen (ultrasound can at times substitute for exploratory surgery); with heart disease when the heartbeat can be observed in its entirety (to test heart valve function); to determine if there is any growth in a body organ; to diagnose prostate disease; to help locate deep-vein thrombosis; to reduce any risks that may accompany amniocentesis by helping to locate the exact position of the fetus and placenta; to detect ectopic (the fetus outside of the uterus) pregnancy.

Normal values: Body organs should appear normal in size and location, and show no evidence of pathology.

Abnormal values: As with several other tests, interpretation depends primarily on the physician's experience rather than on established standards.

UPPER-BOWEL X-RAY, see *Radiography*

UPPER GI SERIES, see *Radiography*

UREA CLEARANCE, see *Creatinine*

UREA NITROGEN (Blood Urea Nitrogen, BUN)

Urea is produced primarily in the liver and is the main nitrogen end product of protein metabolism; it is eliminated by the kidneys into the urine. Normally there is very little urea in the blood. When kidney function is impaired by disease, the normal excretion of urea may be decreased and urea nitrogen in the blood (BUN) is therefore increased. Urea nitrogen varies with dietary protein intake. Blood is collected from a vein and the serum is examined. Urea nitrogen may also be measured in the urine.

A somewhat similar test, called nonprotein nitrogen (NPN), measures all the nitrogen end products in the blood in addition to urea. The NPN is not considered as accurate as the BUN. In fact, many doctors do not consider the BUN alone to be an accurate indicator of kidney function, although it is probably the most commonly ordered kidney test.

When performed: When kidney disease is suspected; when there is an indication that urine production is blocked; when the patient displays mental confusion or disorientation; with evidence of increased pituitary activity (acromegaly); with heart failure; after excessive vomiting, diarrhea, or sweating.

Normal values: BUN normally ranges from 10 to 20 mg per 100 ml of blood. Urine urea is measured over a specific period of time and compared with blood urea to determine normal values.

Abnormal values: BUN is increased (over 30 mg per 100 ml) in kidney disease, fever, starvation (increased breakdown of body protein), internal bleeding, and with the taking of a number of drugs, including certain antibiotics, thiazides (diuretics), methyldopa, salicylates, and chloral hydrate. BUN is decreased in liver disease and with increased pituitary activity. At times, urine urea secretion will be low even if BUN is normal; this is an indication of kidney disease.

URETHRAL OBSTRUCTION, see *Urine Flow Rate*

URIC ACID

Uric acid is an end product of the body's protein metabolism. The amount varies with certain diseases as well as with ingestion of foods such as sweetbreads, liver, anchovies, and sardines. Blood is collected from a vein and the serum is examined for uric acid levels. A 24-hour urine specimen may be collected for measuring uric acid excretion by the kidneys.

When performed: Primarily when there is suspicion of gout; to aid in the diagnosis of leukemia, toxemia of pregnancy, glycogen storage disease, Lesch-Nyhan syndrome (an inherited form of mental retardation), and other conditions where there is destruction of the body's cells.

Normal values: Normal serum uric acid ranges from 2 to 8 mg per 100 ml. Women and children usually have slightly lower values.

Abnormal values: Higher than normal values are usually found with gout, leukemia, heart disease, toxemia of pregnancy, pneumonia, severe kidney damage (which decreases excretion), glycogen storage disease, and Lesch-Nyhan syndrome. Eating certain foods and taking ascorbic acid, salicylates (such as aspirin), theophylline, or thiazides (diuretics) can also increase values. Lower than normal values are usually found in patients taking coumarin products (anticoagulants) and piperazine (worm medicine).

URINALYSIS, see *Urine Examination*

URINARY BLADDER, see *Cystometry*

URINARY 17-KETOSTEROIDS (17-KS), see *Cortisol*

URINARY TRACT CALCULUS

When a stone or calculus (plural: calculi) appears anywhere in the urinary tract (from kidney to bladder), it is essential to analyze the stone to identify its composition. If the primary ingredient of a kidney stone can be determined (identification is possible only in about half of all cases), proper treatment can be started much sooner. Stones may come from eating an excessive amount of food high in **Calcium** and **Oxylates**, metabolic problems, dehydration, excessive vitamin D intake, excessive bed rest, parathyroid gland problems (see **Calcium**), and many other conditions. Nephrocalcinosis (stone formation limited to the kidney) is sometimes visualized by X-ray examination, but in most instances diagnosis is made by identification of the type of crystals in the urine.

When performed: When abdominal, back, or groin pain cannot be diagnosed; when there is evidence of blood in the urine; when the amount of urine is decreased.

Normal values: Normally no crystals should be seen in a microscopic examination of freshly passed urine (at times, certain proteins may crystalize when the urine has cooled to room temperature).

Abnormal values: Pathological crystals have uniquely identifiable shapes and colors. Those that can reflect disease include calcium oxalate (the most common), calcium phosphate, uric acid (not always due to gout), cystine (see **Aminoaciduria**), and tyrosine (usually associated with liver disease). The presence of urinary tract stones more often represents a metabolic or inherited disease than kidney pathology.

URINE CONCENTRATION, see *Mosenthal*

URINE CULTURE, see *Culture*

URINE EXAMINATION

Many urine tests are described under the names of the blood tests that usually accompany them (see, for example, **Albumin/Globulin**; **Glucose**; **Phenylketonuria**). Urine is one of many waste products that indicate the general health of the body in addition to being a specific measure of kidney function. A routine, or screening urine examination usually consists of tests for specific gravity (concentration of solids), protein (albumin), and sugar (glucose); microscopic examination for bacteria, parasites, chemical crystals, and casts (solid matter made up of bacteria, blood cells, pus, protein, etc.); and examination for acid or alkaline reaction, color, odor, and transparency. Many doctors feel the test for protein in the urine is the best single indicator of kidney disease.

Approximately 2 ounces (50 ml) of urine is collected, preferably from an early morning specimen, which contains materials excreted by the kidneys during the night and will usually be of less volume (more concentrated, higher in specific gravity). If the patient drinks an excessive amount of fluids, the amount of urine will increase automatically and the specific gravity will be reduced.

When performed: As a routine screening test to determine kidney function; when liver disease is suspected; as a measure of any disorder of the urinary, cardiovascular, and metabolic systems.

Normal values: Urine should range in color from yellow to light amber and should be clear or transparent. It is normal for early morning urine to have a spicy odor and to be slightly acid. On microscopic examination an occasional red or white blood cell may be seen; the appearance of a few casts after strenuous exercise is still considered normal. Normal specific gravity ranges from 1.010 to 1.025, with a reading toward the higher limit in an early morning specimen.

Abnormal values: With liver disease, certain anemias, melanoma (a form of skin cancer), and excessive intake of vitamins, the urine may have a greenish or brownish tint. A reddish or brownish tint usually indicates the presence of blood.

Whenever the urine is not clear or transparent, more often than not it contains pus, bacteria, blood and/or chemical crystals. Gonorrhea usually causes long, thin, whitish shreds to appear in the urine.

Urine that has an ammonia odor is almost always indicative of some disease condition that causes excessive urine to be retained in the bladder. A sweet or fruity odor is indicative of a dangerous stage of diabetes mellitus.

While the urine normally has a very slight acid reaction, the degree of acidity may increase with kidney disease, heart disease, and diarrhea (from any cause). An alkaline reaction may be seen with certain anemias or various infections and after prolonged vomiting.

Note: The Addis count is a test of urine sediment to determine the amount of protein and the number of red blood cells, white blood cells, casts, and epithelial cells in a 12-hour urine specimen. The Addis count is elevated in kidney disease.

URINE FLOW RATE

The uroflow meter is an electronic device that records the pressure (force), amount, and time required to pass urine. The test is used to determine if any partial obstruction exists in or at the entrance to the urethra (the duct that carries urine from the bladder to outside the body). Reduced flow is most commonly seen in men with prostate problems (an enlarged prostate gland pushes up against the urethra and narrows its diameter). Urine flow is also reduced with old infection, bladder tumors, polyps, urinary tract stones, and nerve diseases that are reflected in lack of normal bladder function.

After drinking at least a quart of liquid four hours before the test, the patient voids (urinates) into a funnel attached to the uroflow meter. Because many patients find it difficult to urinate on command, privacy must be offered to achieve accurate results.

When performed: When a patient complains of pain or difficulty in urinating (getting started, maintaining an even flow) or of frequent urination (usually in very small amounts); when prostatic disease is suspected; following urethral infections, especially gonorrhea; with certain nerve conditions (multiple sclerosis); before and after any surgery in the bladder and urethral area (such as prostate operations).

Normal values: The normal rate is 20 ml per second at maximum flow.

Abnormal values: A rate of less than 10 ml per second is considered abnormal. If the urine flow rate pressure has been measured previously, any relative decrease in that pressure indicates some partial obstruction of the urethra. A decreased amount, or prolonged time for urinating, also indicates obstruction.

URINE TEMPERATURE, see *Body Temperature*

UROBILINOGEN

Urobilinogen comes from bilirubin (a yellow pigment found in bile and after the normal breakdown of red blood cells). The urine normally contains small amounts of urobilinogen, but in certain disease conditions (anemias, liver damage, certain infections) the urobilinogen level in the urine increases. Maximum excretion of urobilinogen usually occurs between one and three in the afternoon. A 2-hour specimen, or a 24-hour sample, may be required for examination.

When performed: When there is suspicion of gall bladder or biliary tract obstruction; with blood or liver problems.

Normal values: One Erlich unit per 100 ml is considered normal in a 2-hour collection of urine preferably collected between 1 and 3 P.M. In a 24-hour sample, excretion of 1 to 4 mg is within the normal range.

Abnormal values: Increased amounts of urobilinogen are found with liver damage and hemolytic anemia. Ingestion of salicylates (such as aspirin) will cause the results of the test to be falsely elevated. Decreased urobilinogen is found in obstructive jaundice. Ingestion of antibiotics may cause the results to be falsely lowered.

UTERINE IRRIGATION, see *Dilatation and Curettage*

VAGINOSCOPY, see *Endoscopy*

VAN DEN BERGH REACTION, see *Bilirubin*

VANILLYMANDELIC ACID, see *Catecholamines*

VARICOSE VEIN INCOMPETENCY, see *Tourniquet Test for Varicose Veins*

VCG, see *Vectorcardiogram*

VDRL, see *Syphilis*

VECTORCARDIOGRAM (VCG)

Sometimes called spatial or three-dimensional electrocardiography, the vector-cardiogram is a somewhat refined version of the standard **Electrocardiogram** (ECG). The VCG shows heart muscle activity or heart damage from two different points in the heart at the same time, thus giving an indication of the *direction* of heart muscle activity as well as its force (contraction and relaxation). The ECG records only the force of heart muscle and from only one location at a time. In the VCG, electrodes are attached to at least four body surfaces (compared with two in the ECG). The electrodes are connected to a measuring instrument with an oscilloscope or cathode-ray tube (similar to a television picture tube), which produces a moving "loop" configuration (in the ECG a line graph on paper is produced). The loop may be observed directly on the oscilloscope, or it may be fed into a computer so that a permanent image can be recorded for analysis at a later time. The image will show the size, shape, and direction of heart muscle activity.

When performed: The VCG is most commonly used to teach physicians how to understand and interpret the ECG; it is also employed when the ECG shows no obvious heart abnormalities but the patient's symptoms indicate a heart problem. Should two or more heart problems be suspected and the ECG show only one, the VCG may reveal the others. It can also aid in determining the extent of heart pathology.

Normal values: There are no standards that can be used for correlation (as exist for the ECG); interpretation of the VCG is based on the doctor's experience with the test.

Abnormal values: By knowing the placement of the electrodes for a particular recording, the physician can determine any abnormalities in the loop formations.

VEIN PRESSURE, see *Blood Pressure*

VEIN SCAN, see *Nuclear Scanning*

VEIN THROMBOSIS, see *Plethysmography*

VENEREAL DISEASE RESEARCH LABORATORY, see *Syphilis*

VENOUS BLOOD PRESSURE, see *Blood Pressure*

VENTILATION, see *Pulmonary Function*

VENTILATION SCAN, see *Nuclear Scanning*

VERTIGO, see *Caloric*

VIRAL PNEUMONIA, see *Agglutination*

VIRUS DISEASE, see *Complement Fixation*

VISION, see *Visual Acuity*

VISUAL ACUITY

Tests of visual acuity (or vision) measure the ability of each eye to perceive the size and shape of an object clearly at standard distances. The tests also measure the ability of both eyes, working together, to discern the distance and depth of objects and their relationship to one another (which object is nearer or further away), called stereopsis or depth perception.

The most common vision test uses the Snellen chart: the patient reads a series of unrelated letters or numbers of various sizes at a distance of 20 feet; for those who cannot read, the letter **E** is used in different sizes and positions (**E**, **ɯ**, **m**). A person with normal vision will easily designate a letter ⅜ inch high from 20 feet away; such visual acuity is recorded as 20/20. The largest letter on the Snellen chart is 3½ inches high; if this is the only letter that a patient can read at a distance of 20 feet, the visual acuity is recorded as 20/200 (reflecting the fact that someone with normal vision could read that letter 200 feet away). The legal definition of blindness is 20/200 vision or worse with the use of the most efficient corrective lens. Normal visual acuity is called emmetropia; a vision defect that can be corrected by the use of lenses is called ametropia.

Myopia, or nearsightedness, is a form of ametropia characterized by difficulty in seeing objects clearly at a distance (usually 20 feet) but being able to read or see objects close up. In hyperopia, sometimes called hypermetropia or farsightedness, patients can see objects clearly at a distance but have difficulty with reading or close work. In presbyopia, usually considered a form of hyperopia as a result of normal aging, the lens of the eye can no longer accommodate (change shape) to focus well on near as well as far objects. With astigmatism, the eye cannot focus properly in certain planes. For example, a person might be able to distinguish all the numbers on a clock except those that are on a line from 11 to 5. Anisometropia is characterized by a difference in visual acuity of the two eyes. This can become a serious problem in children if the eye with the worst vision is not used (amblyopia). Failure to use one eye (sometimes called "lazy eye") can cause **Strabismus**, where the eye no longer focuses on an object and strays outward or inward (cross-eyes). In aphakia, the lens of the eye is absent.

The standard method of vision testing is to have the patient read an eye chart, using trial lenses of different strengths (called refraction) at a distance of 20 feet. Retinoscopy is a much more objective way to test vision, especially with children; it measures the precise way light focuses on the retina in the back of the eye. There are also electronic devices (used mostly by schools, industry, and motor vehicle departments) that can detect most vision problems within minutes. (The Snellen wall chart is best for myopia, but it can easily miss other forms of ametropia.) For more accurate visual acuity testing of patients under 20 years of age whose pupillary muscles are difficult to relax, many doctors use a cyclopegic drug to dilate (relax) those pupillary muscles so that the eye cannot accommodate, or react to light. A simple test for visual acuity involves looking at an object through a pinhole opening. If the object seems much clearer through the pinhole, professional vision testing is indicated.

When performed: Whenever there is difficulty in seeing clearly; as a screening test to detect vision problems before they become serious; as a way of following the course of various diseases such as diabetes; as part of testing candidates for certain occupations (flying).

Normal values: Although 20/20 vision (ability to see a standard-sized letter at 20 feet) is considered normal, up to 20/40 vision without the aid of glasses is still considered satisfactory (a driver's license is usually permitted with this vision). Normally an individual who can see clearly at 20 feet also can read tiny print at a distance of 14 inches. When two objects are in line, a patient with normal vision can discern their relative depth (which one is in front and which one is in back).

Abnormal values: Indications of impaired vision include the inability to read at least 20/40 size letters at a distance of 20 feet (some people may be uncomfortable without 20/20 vision), the inability to read small print at a distance of 14 inches or less, and the inability to perceive the relative depth of objects. Poor visual acuity may be inherited or it may be caused by bodily disease, by many drugs and poisons, and, of course, by problems of the eye itself such as glaucoma, cataract, eye muscle weakness, and any trauma to or around the eye.

Note: Measurement of visual acuity is only one of many different ways to test the eyes. For other, more specific tests, see **Color Blindness**; **Fluorescein Eye Stain**; **Fundoscopy**; **Pupillary Reflex**; **Schirmer's**; **Strabismus**; **Tonometry**; **Visual Field**.

VISUAL FIELD

Central visual field measurements test the eye's ability to see objects over a wide area (peripheral vision) while looking at a specific point. For example, when an individual looks straight ahead, he should still be aware of any object directly at his side. In most instances, an instrument called a perimeter is used to obtain exact measurements (perimetry) of just how far the eye can distinguish objects above, below, and to the side (called field of vision). Perimetry is usually performed after screening tests indicate a visual field defect.

By charting the visual field for each eye, the physician can diagnose various diseases of the brain, the nerves, and the retina. Blind spots (scotoma) can indicate disease; but the eye also has a normal blind spot (where the optic nerve enters the brain). Locating this specific area can verify the test's accuracy as well as detect patients who are faking vision problems. Hemianopia (inability to see the entire visual field) usually indicates a nerve or brain problem.

The simplest way to test visual field is for the doctor and patient to sit three feet apart and each look at the other's nose while the doctor moves his finger above, below, and to the side; both should see the fingertip at the same places. The physician may also mark the patient's visual margins on a tangent screen (a black felt sheet with circles on it) for a permanent record.

When performed: As a routine screening test in any eye examination; when there is suspicion of a brain lesion or an eye defect that cannot be corrected with glasses (such as glaucoma); when inherited eye disease is suspected; in instances of hysteria.

Normal values: The eye, looking directly ahead at a point, should be able to perceive a small (3 mm) spot (it may be a dot on the end of a stick or a tiny light) at an almost 90° angle to the side (away from the nose, toward the temple area of the head). The field of vision normally extends downward past the top of the cheek to an angle of about 65° and upward to an angle of no more than 45°. When looking straight ahead, the eye should also see anything not blocked by the nose. The normal blind spot (which has no visual receptors) is the point where the eye will not see the test spot when looking straight ahead. The patient's perceptions are recorded on a standard visual field chart.

Abnormal values: Any reduction in visual field is indicative of disease. The reduction may be in one direction only, or it may affect the overall field of vision in equal proportions (as with glaucoma or inherited degenerative retinitis). Most abnormalities of the visual field show specific patterns that aid in the diagnosis of a number of eye and brain lesions. Patients can have a markedly diminished field of vision and still have normal **Visual Acuity**.

VISUAL MOTOR PERCEPTION

The Bender Gestalt test of visual motor perception measures how well a child perceives an object and how well he can draw or copy that object. Years of experience have shown that the test is not only an indicator of intelligence (as a predictor of achievement in school; see **Intelligence Quotient**), but can also help diagnose brain injury and mental retardation in children from five to ten years of age.

The child is shown nine geometric and abstract designs and is asked to make a copy of each. The child's response is evaluated for distortions, incompleteness, rotation, or inaccuracies and is scored according to standard values. The age of the child, the time it takes to complete the drawing, and the overall accuracy of the reproduction are taken into account.

When performed: When there is a question of learning ability, especially in a young child about to start school; to assess the possibility of brain damage or mental retardation at the time a child is entering school.

Normal values: The older the child, the less deviation there should be from the original drawing. At the age of five, the child may introduce at least a dozen inaccuracies in copying the drawings. The number of inaccuracies normally decreases to two or less by the time the child reaches ten years of age.

Abnormal values: With brain injury, the child not only makes a great many more errors in copying but introduces many more distortions and has greater problems with integration of shapes. With mental retardation, the child shows no special area of error; the errors are spread uniformly over the test measurements but are markedly increased for the child's age.

VITAL CAPACITY, see *Pulmonary Function*

VITAMIN A, see *Retinol*

VITAMIN B$_1$, see *Thiamin*

VITAMIN B$_2$, see *Riboflavin*

VITAMIN B$_3$, see *Niacin*

VITAMIN B$_6$, see *Pyridoxine*

VITAMIN B$_{12}$, see *Schilling*

VITAMIN C, see *Ascorbic Acid*

VITAMIN D

Vitamin D, which exists in several different forms, is essential to proper development of bones and teeth and proper utilization of calcium in the body. It is found in large amounts in fish (especially fish oils), egg yolks, and butter. Deficiency of vitamin D can cause rickets and osteomalacia (softening of bones, accompanied by pain and muscular weakness). Tooth decay can be caused by too little vitamin D. Excessive intake of vitamin D can cause nausea, loss of appetite, slow growth, and headaches.

The **Alkaline Phosphatase** test is performed to confirm the severity (possible bone involvement) of vitamin D deficiency. Blood is taken from a vein and the serum is examined.

When performed: To diagnose rickets and other bone or teeth abnormalities.

Normal values: Alkaline phosphatase levels range from 2 to 4.5 Bodansky units per 100 ml of serum in adults. The normal range in children is 5 to 15 Bodansky units per 100 ml of serum.

Abnormal values: Values for serum alkaline phosphatase may be increased in vitamin D deficiency and many other conditions (Paget's disease, cancer, hyperparathyroidism, osteogenic sarcoma). An excessive amount of vitamin D can cause decreased alkaline phosphatase values.

VITAMIN E, see *Tocopherols*

VITAMIN K, see *Prothrombin Time*

VMA, see *Catecholamines*

VOICE, see *Hearing Function*

WALDENSTROM'S MACROGLOBULINEMIA, see *Macroglobulin*

WASSERMANN, see *Complement Fixation; Syphilis*

WATER PROVOCATION, see *Tonometry*

WBC, see *White Blood Cell*

WEBER, see *Tuning Fork*

WECHSLER, see *Intelligence Quotient*

WEIL-FELIX, see *Agglutination*

WESTERGREN, see *Sedimentation Rate*

WHISPER, see *Hearing Function*

WHITE BLOOD CELL (Leukocyte, WBC)

The five different types of white blood cells (see **Blood Cell Differential**) are formed and stored in the bone marrow, thymus, lymph glands, and spleen. They are particularly important in fighting infections. The amount of certain kinds of white blood cells usually increases with infection or inflammation in the body, and these blood cells help destroy the causative agents. The white blood cell count is the total of the five kinds of white cells.

A drop of blood from the fingertip, heel, or earlobe (or from blood drawn for other tests) is examined. White blood cells are also searched for in spinal fluid, urine, joint fluid, and mucus. The cells may be counted manually under a microscope, but most often they are counted electronically. (With modern equipment, the cells can be viewed on a TV screen and counted automatically.)

When performed: When infection is suspected; in toxic reactions to certain drugs (sulfa drugs and other antibiotics, analgesics); in toxic reactions to chemicals or poisons (arsenic); in blood disorders, especially leukemias.

Normal values: There should be 5,000 to 10,000 white blood cells per cubic millimeter (cu mm). Children may have higher values.

Abnormal values: The total white blood cell count increases temporarily with most bacterial infections, blood disorders, emotional stress, hemorrhage, rheumatic fever, and burns. A white blood cell count may be falsely elevated when patients feel tense or embarrassed as a result of undergoing an examination. The white blood cell count decreases following ingestion of certain drugs or chemicals, after X-ray treatments, with malaria, typhoid, brucellosis, certain forms of leukemia, and virus and rickettsial infections. The count also decreases when the body produces autoimmune antibody globulins that stop white blood cell production.

Note: The Christmas tree test determines if the white blood cells are performing their function of killing bacteria. A tiny amount of blood is placed on a glass slide stained with a dye. Dead bacteria show up red; live bacteria, green (thus the name Christmas tree). Normally the slide shows very little green color; a lack of red-colored cells indicates the patient's inability to fight infections. The test takes only a few hours (older, similar tests take days).

WHITE BLOOD CELL DIFFERENTIAL, see *Blood Cell Differential*

WIDEL, see *Agglutination*

WINTROBE, see *Sedimentation Rate*

WIRT STEREOPSIS, see *Strabismus*

WOOD ALCOHOL, see *Methanol*

WORM, see *Feces Examination*

WORTH FOUR-DOT, see *Strabismus*

XEROMAMMOGRAPHY, see *Radiography*

X-RAY, see *Radiography*

XYLOSE TOLERANCE

The xylose tolerance test ascertains if the intestines absorb nutrients and medications properly. After fasting for at least eight hours, the patient is given a dose of from 5 to 25 g of D-xylose (a form of sugar in water); too large a dose can cause nausea and diarrhea. All urine excreted over the next five hours is collected and then tested for the D-xylose, which is usually excreted unchanged. The test normally is not performed when the patient is known to have kidney disease; but if necessary then, the level of the sugar can be determined in the blood. At times, antibiotic drugs are given a day or two before the test in order to reduce intestinal bacteria which can interfere with absorption.

When performed: Primarily when there is suspicion of liver or pancreas disease causing a decreased amount of digestive enzyme secretion; when there is unexplained weight loss; when there is suspicion of parasitic diseases; when toxic conditions that affect the intestinal lining (celiac disease, tropical sprue) are suspected; following surgery on the intestines; in certain anemias; when patients take large amounts of drugs such as alcohol, certain antibiotics, and mineral oil.

Normal values: When 5 g of D-xylose are given, the urine should show at least 1.5 g; when 25 g of D-xylose are given, the urine should show more than 3 g. Blood should show at least 20 mg per 100 ml five hours after a 25 g dose.

Abnormal values: D-xylose values are decreased when there is malabsorption in the small intestine. When patients have kidney disease or low thyroid activity, there may be normal absorption by the intestine but decreased urine values. Values may decrease as a patient gets older, but this is not necessarily indicative of disease.

ZINC

A deficiency of zinc, one of the trace elements (a mineral needed in the body in only minute amounts) has been associated with a number of disease conditions; in fact, in virtually all illnesses, blood zinc levels are usually decreased. Zinc is essential to certain enzyme functioning and the prevention or treatment of certain developmental abnormalities such as hypogonadism and growth retardation. One specific dwarfism condition can be corrected by adding zinc to the diet. On a normal diet, the average adult takes in approximately 10 to 15 mg of zinc per day. Oysters, herring, and whole grains are good dietary sources of zinc. Since zinc is necessary to produce testosterone and the testes are known to contain the largest amount of zinc in the body, the "old wives' tale" of oysters being an excellent treatment for male impotence would seem to have some basis in fact.

Blood serum, plasma, urine, and even hair are examined for zinc levels. For confirmation of a specific zinc deficiency problem, supplementary zinc is prescribed and the patient is clinically observed for reversal of symptoms.

When performed: When symptoms of abnormalities in taste and smell suggest a zinc deficiency; with prostate disease.

Normal values: Normally the level of zinc found in blood serum is 90 to 110 mcg per 100 ml; 0.5 mg per day is excreted in the urine.

Abnormal values: Lower than normal values of zinc are found in alcoholism, during pregnancy, after a heart attack, after surgery when there is poor wound healing, in liver disease, infections, cancers, and prostate problems. Certain hormones may also lower zinc levels.

Higher than normal levels of zinc are found in patients who inherit a tendency toward hyperzincemia and also in certain metal workers (usually from breathing zinc fumes); an excess amount of zinc can cause drowsiness, dizziness and muscular incoordination.

ZOLLINGER-ELLISON SYNDROME, see *Gastrin*

ZUNG SELF-RATING DEPRESSION SCALE, see *Depression*

Appendix: GENERAL MEDICAL CONDITIONS AND RELATED TESTS

When a patient is ill, certain tests are routinely performed to aid in diagnosis and to follow the progress of treatment. The list below provides a general idea of some tests that may be indicated in various general medical conditions. Not all the tests listed are always utilized. The specific tests recommended by a physician will depend on the patient's medical history, symptoms, signs and the results of the doctor's physical examination. Details of each test, and its disease specificity, are found in the individual test listings.

ADRENAL DISEASE

Aldosterone, Blood Cell Differential, Blood Pressure, Calcium, Carbon Dioxide, Catecholamines, Chloride, Cortisol, Estrogen, Magnesium, Mosenthal, pH, Potassium, Renin, Sodium

ALCOHOLISM

Albumin/Globulin, Alcohol, Alcoholism, Aldolase, Ammonia, Ascorbic Acid, Barbiturates, Blood Cell Differential, Carcinoembryonic Antigen, Cerebellum, Creatine Phosphokinase, Folates, Glucose, Lipids, Magnesium, Methanol, Niacin, Occult Blood, Osmolality, Schilling, Sweat, Uric Acid, Xylose Tolerance, Zinc

ALLERGY

Blood Cell Differential, Carbon Dioxide, Complement, Culture, Feces Examination, Fungus, Immunoglobulin, Pulmonary Function, RAST, Skin Reaction, Sputum, Tartrazine Sensitivity

ANEMIA

Agglutination, Aldolase, Alkaline Phosphatase, Bence-Jones Protein, Bilirubin, Bleeding and Clotting Time, Blood Cell Differential, Bone Marrow, Calcitonin, Caloric, Capillary Fragility, Copper, Feces Examination, Folates, Gastric Analysis, Gastrin, Glucose-6 Phosphate Dehydrogenase, HAM, Haptoglobin, Hematocrit, Hemoglobin, HL-A Antigen, Icterus Index, Iron, Lactic Acid, Lactic Dehydrogenase, Macroglobulin, Malaria, Occult Blood, Oxygen, Platelet Count, Red Blood Cell, Reticulocyte Count, Riboflavin, Schilling, Tocopherols, Typing and Cross Matching, Urine Examination, Urobilinogen, White Blood Cell

ARTHRITIS (AND JOINT DISEASE)

Antinuclear Antibodies, Complement, C-Reactive Protein, HL-A Antigen, Radiography, Salicylates, Sedimentation Rate, Synovial Fluid, Thoracentesis, Uric Acid

BIRTH DEFECTS

Alpha Fetoprotein, Aminoaciduria, Amniocentesis, Cerebrospinal Fluid, Chromatin, Creatine Phosphokinase, Ketones, Lipids, Phenylketonuria, Phytohemagglutinin, Placental Lactogen, Sweat, Uric Acid, Visual Motor Perception

BONE DISEASE

Acid Phosphatase, Alkaline Phosphatase, Calcium, Hydroxyproline, Nuclear Scanning, Phosphorus, Radiography, Retinol, Synovial Fluid, Vitamin D

BRAIN DISEASE

Caloric, Carbon Dioxide, Cerebellum, Cerebrospinal Fluid, Chlorides, Cognitive Capacity Screening, Computerized Tomography, Drug Monitoring, Electroencephalogram, Electromyography, Exophthalmometer, Facial Recognition, Fundoscopy, Glucose, Hearing Function, Intelligence Quotient, Ketones, Lactic Acid, Language Function, Manganese, Mercury, Methanol, Motor Development, Niacin, Nuclear Scanning, pH, Phenylketonuria, Porphyrins, Potassium, Prolactin, Pulmonary Function, Pupillary

Reflex, Radiography, Reflex, Salicylates, Sensory, Smell Function, Strabismus, Syphilis, Taste, Tuning Fork, Visual Acuity, Visual Field, Visual Motor Perception, Zinc

CANCER

Acid Phosphatase, Aldolase, Aldosterone, Alkaline Phosphatase, Alpha Fetoprotein, Ascorbic Acid, Bence-Jones Protein, Bilirubin, Biopsy, Blood Cell Differential, Calcitonin, Carcinoembryonic Antigen, Cerebrospinal Fluid, Complement, Computerized Tomography, C-Reactive Protein, Cytology, Dilatation and Curettage, Endoscopy, Estrogen Receptor, Exophthalmometer, Feces Examination, Fibrinogen, Fundoscopy, Gastric Analysis, Gastrin, Glucagon, Haptoglobin, Immunoglobulin, Insulin, Iron, Isocitric Dehydrogenase, Lactic Dehydrogenase, Lipase, Macroglobulin, Melanogen-Melanin, Occult Blood, Porphyrins, Radiography, Red Blood Cell, Schiller, Sedimentation Rate, Serotonin, Sputum, Thermography, Thoracentesis, Urine Flow Rate, Vitamin D

DIABETES

Blood Pressure, Chloride, C-Peptide, Finger Wrinkle, Fundoscopy, Glucagon, Glucose, Glycohemoglobin, Growth Hormone, Insulin, Ketones, Lactic Acid, Osmolality, Potassium, Sodium, Tonometry, Urine Examination, Visual Acuity

EAR DISEASE

Caloric, Hearing Function, Radiography, Salicylates, Tuning Fork, Tympanometry

EDEMA

Albumin/Globulin, Aldosterone, Computerized Tomography, Mosenthal, Osmolality, Phenolsulfonphthalein, Plethysmography, Pulmonary Function, Sodium, Thiamin, Thoracentesis, Urine Examination

EYE DISEASE

Color Blindness, Exophthalmometer, Fluorescein Eye Stain, Fundoscopy, Methanol, Pupillary Reflex, Radiography, Reflex, Retinol, Riboflavin, Schirmer's, Strabismus, Tensilon, Tonometry, Ultrasound, Visual Acuity, Visual Field, Visual Motor Perception

GALL BLADDER DISEASE

Alkaline Phosphatase, Amylase, Bilirubin, Bromsulphalein Retention, Cephalin Flocculation, Computerized Tomography, Endoscopy, Feces Examination, Icterus Index, Leucine Aminopeptidase, Radiography, Ultrasound, Urobilinogen

GASTROINTESTINAL DISEASE

Amylase, Bicarbonate, Carbon Dioxide, Carcinoembryonic Antigen, Chloride, Computerized Tomography, Cytology, Endoscopy, Feces Examination, Folates, Gastric Analysis, Gastrin, Lactose Tolerance, Lipase, Mercury, Mononucleosis, Niacin, Occult Blood, Oxalate, pH, Porphyrins, Potassium, Pyridoxine, Radiography, Retinol, Schilling, Serotonin, Taste, Ultrasound, Xylose Tolerance

HEART (CIRCULATION) DISEASE

Aldolase, Antistreptolysin O Titer, Apexcardiogram, Ballistocardiogram, Blood Pressure, Circulation Time, Cooper, C-Reactive Protein, Creatine Phosphokinase, Digitalis Toxicity, Drug Monitoring, Echocardiogram, Electrocardiogram, Endoscopy, Fundoscopy, Glutamic Oxalacetic Transaminase, Hydroxybutyric Dehydrogenase, Jenkins Activity Survey, Lactic Dehydrogenase, Lipoproteins, Nuclear Scanning, Oxygen, Phonocardiogram, Platelet Count, Plethysmography, Potassium, Prothrombin Time, Pulmonary Function, Pulse Analysis, Radarkymogram, Radiography, Sedimentation Rate, Selenium, Sodium, Syphilis, Systolic Time Intervals, Thermography, Thiamin, Tourniquet Test for Varicose Veins, Ultrasound, Urea Nitrogen, Urine Examination, Vectorcardiogram

HEMORRHAGE

Bleeding and Clotting Time, Capillary Fragility, Computerized Tomography, Endoscopy, Fibrinogen, Hematocrit, Hemoglobin, Macroglobulin, Partial Thromboplastin Time, Platelet Count, Prothrombin Time, Radiography, Red Blood Cell, Reticulocyte Count, Synovial Fluid, Typing and Cross Matching, White Blood Cell

HIGH BLOOD PRESSURE

Aldosterone, Blood Pressure, Fundoscopy, Phenolsulfonphthalein, Radiology, Renin, Rollover, Sodium

INFECTION

Agglutination, Albumin/Globulin, Aldolase, Amylase, Antinuclear Antibodies, Antistreptolysin O Titer, Ascorbic Acid, Australian Antigen, Blood Cell Differential, Bone Marrow, Cerebrospinal Fluid, Chloride, Complement, Complement Fixation, Copper, C-Reactive Protein, Culture, Dilatation and Curettage, Endoscopy, Feces Examination, Fungus, Gastric Analysis, Gastrin, Glutamic Oxalacetic Transaminase, Gram Stain, Growth Hormone, HAM, Haptoglobin, Herpes, HL-A Antigen, Immunoglobulin, Iron, Kveim, Lactic Dehydrogenase, Macroglobulin, Malaria, Mononucleosis, Oxalate, Phytohemagglutinin, Platelet Count, Plethysmography, Pulmonary Function, Pupillary Reflex, Pyridoxine, Radiography, RAST, Red Blood Cell, Reflex, Riboflavin, Scabies, Schiller, Schilling, Schirmer's, Sedimentation Rate, Sensory, Skin Reaction, Smell Function, Sputum, Sweat, Synovial Fluid, Syphilis, Thoracentesis, Tonometry, Urea Nitrogen, Urine Examination, Urine Flow Rate, White Blood Cell, Xylose Tolerance, Zinc

INJURY

Aldolase, Carbon Dioxide, Cerebellum, Cerebrospinal Fluid, Computerized Tomography, Creatine Phosphokinase, Electroencephalogram, Electromyography, Feces Examination, Fundoscopy, Haptoglobin, Hearing Function, Hemoglobin, Hydroxyproline, Impotence, pH, Phosphorus, Platelet Count, Plethysmography, Pulmonary Function, Radiography, Synovial Fluid, Taste, Tonometry, Ultrasound, White Blood Cell

KIDNEY AND URINARY TRACT DISEASE

Albumin/Globulin, Aldosterone, Amylase, Antistreptolysin O Titer, Bicarbonate, Blood Pressure, Calcitonin, Chloride, Cholinesterase, Complement, Computerized Tomography, Congo Red, Creatinine, Cystometry, Cytology, Endoscopy, Glucose, HAM, HL-A Antigen, Immunoglobulin, Lactic Acid, Mercury, Mosenthal, Nuclear Scanning, Occult Blood, Osmolality, Oxalate, pH, Phenolsulfonphthalein, Phosphorus, Porphyrins, Potassium, Radiography, Red Blood Cell, Renin, Sedimentation Rate, Sodium, Ultrasound, Urea Nitrogen, Uric Acid, Urinary Tract Calculus, Urine Examination

LEUKEMIA

Alkaline Phosphatase, Bleeding and Clotting Time, Blood Cell Differential, Bone Marrow, Copper, Hemoglobin, Immunoglobulin, Lysozyme, Macroglobulin, Platelet Count, Uric Acid, White Blood Cell

LIVER DISEASE

Albumin/Globulin, Alcohol, Alcoholism, Aldolase, Aldosterone, Alkaline Phosphatase, Alpha Fetoprotein, Ammonia, Australian Antigen, Barbiturates, Bilirubin, Bleeding and Clotting Time, Bromsulphalein Retention, Carcinoembryonic Antigen, Cephalin Flocculation, Cholesterol, Cholinesterase, Complement, Computerized Tomography, Copper, Endoscopy, Estrogen, Fibrinogen, Glucose, Glutamic Oxalacetic Transaminase, Haptoglobin, Icterus Index, Isocitric Dehydrogenase, Lactic Dehydrogenase, Leucine Aminopeptidase, Macroglobulin, Mosenthal, Nuclear Scanning, pH,

Porphyrins, Prothrombin Time, Radiography, Selenium, Sweat, Taste, Thymol Turbidity, Ultrasound, Urea Nitrogen, Uric Acid, Urinary Tract Calculus, Urine Examination, Urobilinogen, Zinc

LUNG DISEASE

Aldolase, Antinuclear Antibodies, Bicarbonate, Blood Pressure, Carbon Dioxide, Carcinoembryonic Antigen, Cholinesterase, Circulation Time, C-Reactive Protein, Cytology, Echocardiogram, Endoscopy, Fungus, Lactic Dehydrogenase, Methanol, Nuclear Scanning, Oxygen, pH, Phytohemagglutinin, Plethysmography, Pulmonary Function, Radiography, Red Blood Cell, Salicylates, Sputum, Taste, Thoracentesis, Tocopherols

MUSCLE DISEASE

Aldolase, Antinuclear Antibodies, Carbon Dioxide, Catecholamines, Cerebellum, Complement, Creatine Phosphokinase, Creatinine, Electromyography, Glutamic Oxalacetic Transaminase, HAM, HL-A Antigen, Magnesium, Mercury, Motor Development, pH, Phosphorus, Potassium, Pulmonary Function, Reflex, Selenium, Sensory, Strabismus, Tensilon, Thiamin, Tuning Fork, Vitamin D

NERVE DISEASE

Catecholamines, Cerebellum, Cholinesterase, Electroencephalogram, Electromyography, Finger Wrinkle, Mononucleosis, Phosphorus, Pupillary Reflex, Pyridoxine, Reflex, Riboflavin, Selenium, Sensory, Sweat, Syphilis, Taste, Thermography, Thiamin, Tuning Fork, Urine Flow Rate, Zinc

NUTRITIONAL DISORDERS

Albumin/Globulin, Alkaline Phosphatase, Ascorbic Acid, Blood Cell Differential, Carbon Dioxide, Congo Red, Copper, Feces Examination, Fibrinogen, Folates, Gastric Analysis, Gastrin, Glucagon, Glucose, Glycohemoglobin, Hematocrit, Hemoglobin, Hydroxyproline, Iron, Ketones, Lactic Dehydrogenase, Lactose Tolerance, Lipids, Magnesium, Niacin, Osmolality, Oxalate, Phosphorus, Phytohemagglutinin, Prothrombin Time, Pyridoxine, Retinol, Schilling, Sweat, Tocopherols, Urea Nitrogen, Vitamin D, Xylose Tolerance

PANCREATIC DISEASE

Amylase, C-Peptide, Creatinine, Feces Examination, Glucagon, Glucose, Insulin, Lipase, Nuclear Scanning, Phytohemagglutinin, Radiography, Sodium, Ultrasound

PARATHYROID DISEASE

Alkaline Phosphatase, Calcium, Magnesium, Phosphorus, Radiography, Vitamin D

PITUITARY DISEASE

Cortisol, Estrogen, Growth Hormone, Mosenthal, Prolactin, Radiography, Testis Function, Thyroid Function, Urea Nitrogen

POISONING (INCLUDING DRUG ABUSE)

Agglutination, Aldolase, Barbiturates, Bicarbonate, Bilirubin, Blood Cell Differential, Bone Marrow, Bromides, Calcium, Carbon Dioxide, Cerebellum, Cholinesterase, Digitalis Toxicity, Drug Monitoring, Hemoglobin, Lactic Acid, Lead, Lipase, Lithium, Mercury, Oxalate, Oxygen, pH, Porphyrins, Pulmonary Function, Pupillary Reflex, Red Blood Cell, Reflex, Salicylates, Sedimentation Rate, Tartrazine Sensitivity, Uric Acid, Urine Examination, White Blood Cell

PREGNANCY

Agglutination, Aldosterone, Alpha Antitrypsin, Alpha Fetoprotein, Amniocentesis, Blood Pressure, Copper, Estrogen, Folates, Hemoglobin, Isocitric Dehydrogenase, Ketones, Lactic Dehydrogenase, Nuclear Scanning, Placental Lactogen, Pregnancy, Prolactin, Radiography, Rollover, Uric Acid, Urine Examination

SKIN DISEASE

Aminoaciduria, Antinuclear Antibodies, Ascorbic Acid, Biopsy, Cholesterol, Cholinesterase, Complement, Congo Red, Fibrinogen, Fungus, Glucagon, Herpes, HL-A Antigen, Immunoglobulin, Iron, Melanogen-Melanin, Niacin, Phytohemagglutinin, Platelet Count, Porphyrins, Pyridoxine, Riboflavin, Scabies, Sedimentation Rate, Selenium, Sensory, Skin Reaction, Sweat, Synovial Fluid, Syphilis, Tartrazine Sensitivity, Thermography, Tocopherols, Tourniquet

SEXUAL PROBLEMS

Acid Phosphatase, Body Temperature, Chromatin, Cortisol, Dilatation and Curettage, Endoscopy, Estrogen, Fungus, Growth Hormone, Herpes, Impotence, Plethysmography, Radiography, Retinol, Rubin, Schiller, Semen, Tackmeter, Testis Function, Thermography, Zinc

THYROID DISEASE

Basal Metabolic Rate, Blood Cell Differential, Blood Pressure, Calcitonin, Calcium, Cholesterol, Creatine Phosphokinase, Exophthalmometer, Magnesium, Nuclear Scanning, Radiography, Sedimentation Rate, Sweat, Thyroid Function, Tonometry, Ultrasound

MEASUREMENTS: EQUIVALENCY CHART
MASS OR SOLID SUBSTANCE MEASUREMENTS

kg	kilogram	1000 g; 2 pounds, 3 ounces; 2.2 lb; 35.27 oz
g	gram	1000 mg; 0.035 oz; $1/30$ oz (28.35 g = 1 oz); 15½ grains (weight of a paper clip)
mg	milligram	1000 μg; 0.001 g; 0.000035 oz; 1/65 grain (2 particles of table salt)
μg , mcg	microgram	1000 ng; 1/1000000 g (one millionth of a gram)
ng	nanogram	1000 pg; 1/1000000000 g (one billionth of a gram)*
pg	picogram	1/1000000000000 g (one trillionth of a gram)* *

* Drugs such as LSD and amphetamines can cause a toxic or even fatal reaction in such small doses that they are measured in nanograms. Cardiac glycosides (such as Digoxin and Digitoxin) and other drugs that produce a therapeutic effect in very small amounts are also measured in nanograms; in some patients a toxic overdose can be caused by a rise of only one nanogram in the blood.

* * Many hormone tests are reported in picograms.

LIQUID MEASUREMENTS

L	liter	1000 ml; 1.06 qts; 1 qt, 2 oz; 33.81 oz
dl	deciliter	100 ml; 3.4 oz (gradually replacing 100 ml in reported test values)
ml	milliliter	.001 L; 1/1000 L (one thousandth of a liter); (5 ml = 1 teaspoon; 30 ml = 1 oz)*
μl	microliter	1/1000000 L (one millionth of a liter)

* At times, cc (cubic centimeter) is used inaccurately for, or interchangeably with, ml; cc is more properly a measure of area rather than of volume or quantity of liquid.